Long Time, No See

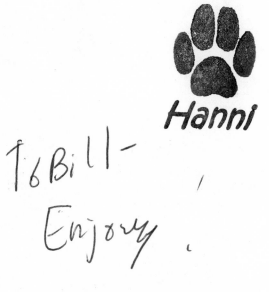

Hanni

To Bill—

Enjoy.

Long Time, No See

Beth Finke

UNIVERSITY OF ILLINOIS PRESS

URBANA AND CHICAGO

Library of Congress
Cataloging-in-Publication Data
Finke, Beth, 1958–
Long time, no see / Beth Finke.
p.   cm.
ISBN 0-252-02827-9 (cloth : alk. paper)
1. Finke, Beth, 1958–   .
2. People with visual disabilities—United
States—Biography.
3. Diabetics—United States—Biography.
I. Title.
HV1792.F56A3   2003
362.4'1'092—dc21   2002012713
 [B]

To Mike, Gus, and Flo
my sources of inspiration

Contents

Long Time, No See

Prologue:
The Lights Go Out

"How's your *right* eye doing?" Dr. Ernest asked as he rolled his stool from the examination chair.

When I lifted my head to respond, amoeba-like blobs swirled in front of me, as if I was peering out from inside a Christmas snow globe. I had learned to keep my head still, working around these floaters whenever I really wanted to see. Waiting for them to settle, I considered my answer.

My walking stick had become a regular accessory. I used it like a white cane to judge steps and curbs on my walk to work. Just a few days earlier at the office I'd spilled a coffee filter full of grounds, having misjudged the position of its slot on the coffee maker. I sat inches away from my computer screen and still couldn't always make out the words. And my boss had just told me I wouldn't be attending an upcoming national conference because, as she put it, "You'll embarrass the office."

"Not so well," I finally answered, with understatement that now seems comical.

It was a gray Chicago winter morning in 1985, and I was at the University of Illinois eye clinic. My left eye had suddenly gone from bad to useless despite the fact that, nearly every Friday for months, Mike had driven me the 150 miles from Champaign for exams and laser treatments.

I first met Dr. Ernest long before my vision troubles began. Because I had lacked a full-time job with health benefits, I eagerly enrolled in his National Institutes of Health study, which focused on eye disease caused by diabetes. Now, two years later, health insurance was no longer an issue; still, maintaining access to specialists like him was worth the hassle.

The visits had become routine: the couple of hours on the road, the dull hues of the clinic waiting room. After I checked in, a nurse would come with eye drops. We'd wait for my pupils to dilate, Mike flipping through the same out-of-date sports magazine, both of us sipping bitter coffee from Styrofoam cups. Finally I'd be ushered into an exam room and inspected. Depending on what the doctor saw, I'd have laser treatments. Or not.

I'd had so many treatments that even they had become old hat. I was positioned in a chair with footrests and big padded arms; the doctor swiveled out the laser unit until it aligned with the eye being treated.

"Look left," he said. "Now right . . . and down . . . and right again . . . *hold still.*"

Then a pause, the flash of xenon, blue and green.

"Now look up . . . a little to the right. Yes, *there.*"

Another pause, another flash.

For a while these laser treatments halted, or at least slowed, the deterioration of my vision.

But then my left eye went black. Dr. Ernest had suggested a Saturday appointment so we would have time to discuss treatment options. (On weekdays he was continually interrupted, and each time I left his office, other doctors and students were clustered outside, each with "one quick question.")

There was even time for pleasantries. We all had a laugh when the doctor, who'd grown up on a Wisconsin dairy farm and retained his down-to-earth sensibilities, told a story about life in the tony suburb where his family lived. His daughter's elementary school soccer team had lost their last couple of games.

"Quite a scandal," he said sarcastically. "You know what they did? They brought in a sports psychologist. A sports psychologist for an elementary school soccer team!"

I'd been focusing on his face as he told this story. My amoebas and spiders had settled, and I could see well enough to notice him rolling his eyes in disgust. We were all grateful for this non-medical moment.

But in an instant his demeanor and voice changed dramatically. He brought out a model of the human eye, a plastic globe about the size of a softball. He popped the top off and pointed to the inner wall of the sphere and started giving what was essentially the same mini-lecture he'd given when I first started seeing him. Given my current condition, I didn't mind hearing it again.

The retina is the light-sensitive film of cells lining the back of the eye; in its center is an area called the macula where the cells are particularly dense. "The whole area surrounding the retina and macula is rich in blood vessels," he explained. "The longer a patient survives diabetes, the more likely it is that these vessels will become clogged. Glucose—sugar in the bloodstream—combines with some of the proteins that make up the outer coating of your red blood cells, and that makes them sticky."

That was the villainous diabetic retinopathy in a nutshell. In the past, when I'd had this explained to me, I had cringed to recall all the times I'd been less than careful with my insulin. Now those recollections hit me like arrows through my chest.

New blood vessels compensate for the blocked ones, he went on. The problem is that they grow so thick they can keep the light from reaching the retina; they can even tear the retina off the back of the eye. "To make matters worse, they're very thin walled and easily damaged, which means they tend to hemorrhage." He paused a moment for this information to soak in.

"Until now," he said, "laser treatments have been enough to stop your hemorrhaging and control the growth of the new vessels. But now the vessels are growing too fast and bleeding so much that we can no longer see what we're doing in there. If we continue the laser treatments in your left eye, it will be like trying to do the surgery blindfolded."

He laid out my options. I could wait and see if my left eye, the one I couldn't see out of at all, would clear on its own. If it did, the specialist could look inside to determine whether more laser treatments were called for. Or I could have something called a vitrectomy. He asked me what I knew about this surgery.

I had read a pamphlet about it. "They cut open the eye and replace all the bloody fluid with saline solution, right?"

He fixed me in his gaze. "It sounds pretty straightforward in the brochures, but vitrectomy is still a dicey proposition. It's very delicate and not always successful. As long as we're still able, we'd like to avoid major surgery and keep on with laser treatments."

Either way, my right eye would continue to be treated periodically with lasers, as long as the specialist could see inside it well enough.

At first, I leaned toward having the vitrectomy—and right away. At least we'd be *doing* something. I was tired of waiting. And waiting was worse than maddening; it was downright risky. The longer we waited, the more damage those blood vessels could do to my retina.

On the other hand, whereas laser treatments were done on an outpatient basis, a vitrectomy was major surgery with general anesthesia. And it didn't always work.

Mike and I looked at each other. We decided to wait. At least for a while.

That I was even considering major eye surgery was a function of how weary I was, having lived in the awkward and dangerous purgatory between being sighted and being blind.

It had been bad enough with two semi-functional eyes. With only one, I grew more and more dependent on those around me, especially Mike. Driving was out of the question. Even walking around town alone had become tricky, and I could no longer ride the beautiful blue Peugeot bicycle Mike had given me the previous Christmas. Confident the lasers would restore me to full sight, I'd stowed the bike in our shed until that day. In the meantime, Mike chauffeured me to work. Even if I was game to walk on my own, he constantly worried about me and urged me to accept the rides.

I was twenty-six years old then. I loved my job, which involved advising American students on their best options for overseas study and helping foreign students adjust to life in the United States. I attended conferences and even visited overseas universities now and then.

My co-workers and our friends in Champaign-Urbana knew Mike and I had been traveling back and forth to Chicago for eye treatments, but they knew little else. It wasn't that we were secretive; we just didn't think the situation was grave enough to dwell on. We felt sure the treatments would eventually work and that soon I'd be back to seeing well. And when we weren't at the clinic in Chicago, the last thing we wanted to talk about was my eyes. We wanted to enjoy ourselves in our old normal ways.

Going to sporting events, for example. It was actually at a University of Illinois basketball game that friends who hadn't seen us in a while began to notice my struggles. That winter we had lucked upon some great seats, very near the court. But being close made it all the harder for me to adjust my eyes fast enough. Mike learned to do a great play-by-play to keep me involved.

"You've never needed Mike to explain basketball strategy before," our friend Russ remarked one night. I just smiled. After that game, as Mike held my hand and coached me up the Assembly Hall steps, I think Russ caught on.

We still went to movies, which were easier than basketball games.

Sure, there was a lot of movement, but it happened on one well-defined surface. I could sit still, find a gap through the blobs in my eye, then stare at the center of the screen, where most of the action was. I saw Prince's body in *Purple Rain*, Darryl Hannah's fin in *Splash*. I remember the round hat on the little boy in *Witness*. Other movies were harder. *The Cotton Club* and *Amadeus* were way too dark. My night vision had been greatly diminished by hemorrhages and laser beams; dull or poorly lighted things became invisible to me. Until the screen lit up, I was totally blind in a movie theater. Again Mike used his new expertise as a guide, directing me to a seat, warning me where the steps were. For most movies I didn't need his play-by-play; I could usually figure out who was saying what to whom.

Except for the time we went to the foreign movie, an act that still falls near the top of my "What Were We Thinking?" list. I know some French and German, but I couldn't concentrate on the dialogue while laboring to see. And the subtitles scampered by too quickly. We walked out on *La Cage aux Folles*, the first time I'd ever left a movie before it was over.

Entertaining myself was particularly difficult. I had never liked TV much, even when I could see well; struggling to watch it seemed absurd. I used to spend hours at our upright piano, playing Broadway tunes and pop songs. But now, unable to read the sheet music, I was limited to plunking out simple pieces with a finger or two. Playing became downright depressing, a step backwards.

Mike helped the cause with a Christmas gift. This year, instead of a bicycle, he gave me a second-hand fiddle. It was a struggle to hold it at the proper angle, pressing strings down at precise points and keeping the bow right over the f-holes. But after a few lessons I was able to scratch out a tune. What a relief it was, learning to do something new, something difficult, when I was starting to fail at simple things, like stepping over curbs. Or making the morning coffee. Or reading.

Moving my eyes to read words on a page shifted the blobs in my narrow field of vision, often obscuring the very text I was trying to read. I was determined to continue reading newspapers, spreading the sheets on the floor and hovering over them like a robot: I held my head still while moving my trunk back and forth, scanning the pages. I checked out large-print books from the library but soon found them of no help: wider words required more eye movement, which meant more blob movement. Commercial talking books weren't yet popular in 1984, and I had yet to learn about the Library of Congress Talking Book Program. So the only books I bothered with were those I had to read for work.

— —

At the office I managed to hold my own in terms of my counseling duties, but I needed more and more help doing simple things like running the copier. My office mates chipped in gladly, but I grew tired of searching for clear lines of sight through the red and black kaleidoscope of my right eye. I was sick of bruising my hips on the office furniture, tired of worrying about what I might or might not see when I awoke each morning.

There was one bright spot: an organization had invited me to visit Denmark and the Soviet Union to observe their exchange programs. I was allowed to bring a guest. Because Mike had studied Russian in college, he was keen on coming along.

After we scheduled the trip, we had second thoughts. It was the first time we confronted the cold, clinical facts in a practical way. If I might really lose my sight, we figured we should go now, while I could still see. But what if skipping the checkups and laser treatments would hurt my cause?

And so we bailed out.

Five months passed and my left eye had failed to clear. The decision to have the vitrectomy became academic.

Surgery day dawned crisp and clear in March 1985. The pre-op folderol had been accomplished the previous day. We walked through the same doors we had opened every Friday for months, although today I had deprived myself of breakfast, as instructed. Neither had I taken my morning insulin—for the first morning in almost twenty years. Though my brain knew it made sense because I wouldn't eat that day, my soul was scared.

Mike held my hand through everything, letting go only when I was transferred onto a gurney and wheeled into the OR. I had already been given a sedative, and the last thing I remember as I lost consciousness was Mike's caress.

Mike's hand was there when I woke up, too—only this time he was touching my forehead. I was barfing my guts out, and he was doing his best to keep my hair out of the way. I was on my stomach, and not all of my vomit was landing in the nifty kidney-shaped bowl. My body ached, my eye was patched, and my aim was terribly off.

"I love you," Mike whispered. The idea that he could love a hospital-gown-clad woman adorned with an eye patch and vomit made me want to laugh. I tried but dry-heaved instead. Never before had I felt this miserable.

Nurses came to clean up the mess. I turned my head away and was instantly scolded: "*No!*" one of them said. No turning.

An air bubble had been placed inside my eyeball to hold the retina in place as I healed. It would gradually shrink by assimilation and my retina would stay where it belonged, but I had to remain face down at all times. My life was like a sketch from *Monty Python's Flying Circus.* Even trudging to the bathroom, I had to bow my head. While I visited with Mike, talked to the doctors and nurses, answered the phone, listened to the TV, ate, drank, and took sponge baths, I faced the floor.

Reading and writing were nearly impossible. Sleeping face down on my little hemorrhoid pillow was the hardest. Inevitably I would roll my head and awake in panic, search for the doughnut and smash my face into it as fast as I could. *Oh no, I've blown it!* I'd think, wondering if I'd already done the damage. Afraid even to doze, rattled by worries, I'd stay awake until the resident came at 5:30 to take me to the exam room.

There I enjoyed five minutes of bliss as I lifted my head onto the chin rest. I actually liked the ache in my underused neck muscles and anticipated the sting that came when the bandages were removed. The resident would ask me to look in all directions, inspecting my eye. "The bubble any smaller?" I'd ask every day, knowing that when it was gone I'd be able to lift my head again, permanently. For more than a month I got the same answer: "It's smaller, but still there."

Typically, at this point the surgeon would arrive, scope my eye, point some things out to the resident, tell me it was still hard to see much, then leave.

Mike always broke the visiting-hour rules by staying late on Saturday night, but Sundays he had to leave earlier to drive back to Champaign. I cried every Sunday after he left. I wanted to get in that car with him, take up life in our crummy little campus apartment again, sleep in my own bed with him, and go back to work on Monday like everybody else.

Mike was the only outsider who saw me during my first recovery. I had asked him to tell family and friends not to phone or visit, to explain that the practicalities of locating the phone or relating to people with my head in a hemorrhoid pillow were too daunting.

Our friends in Champaign, 150 miles away, easily respected my wishes. Mike acted as my press agent, taking phone calls and answering questions. On weekends I'd beg for details—Where'd you go this week? What all did you talk about? Did you run into anyone I know? I was spellbound by his stories; they spirited me away.

As for my family, I am the youngest of seven. Many of my siblings and nieces and nephews are far flung, but my mom and two of my sisters lived in Chicago suburbs. The University of Illinois Eye and Ear Infirmary wasn't far from them, but it was on Chicago's West Side, not far from the Robert Taylor housing projects made infamous in Alex Kotlowitz's *There Are No Children Here*. My mom marveled that Mike and I dared to walk the sidewalks of this neighborhood, much less to eat in its restaurants. She or my sisters would have risked visiting only if my surgery were a grave crisis; I convinced them that it wasn't.

Frankly, I was grateful that none of them showed up. Their absence reassuringly confirmed my rather circular logic: because they weren't there, my situation wasn't dire.

So Mike provided my only relief, my only messenger from outside the hospital.

"How are you doing?" I asked during one of his weekend visits. "I mean, really, how are you *managing*?"

"It's easy," he said.

Too bad my head was stuck in that pillow. The look on my face would have given him a laugh.

"The way I figure it, there's no choice: We have to do whatever it takes to save your vision. That's what I mean by easy."

I nodded into the pillow.

"But it all feels pretty unnatural," Mike finally admitted. "I guess I have a sort of wartime mentality about it. We just have to march."

One of Mike's visits happened to coincide with the Chicago White Sox home opener. Our pal Russ and his office mates were going, and they'd invited Mike. I practically had to pry this from him, but when I did, I urged him, cajoled him to go. You only get so many home openers. After much hand wringing, he went. It was good for both of us; he came back energized, bearing new tales.

━━━   ▬

We marched through a month of hemorrhoid pillows, morning eye exams, prednisone pills and weekday absences from each other—only to find that we'd lost the war. The surgery had failed.

"We can see inside your eye now," I remember the surgeon telling me after my exam one morning.

I was elated. *Finally.*

"The gas bubble has deflated," he continued, ignoring my happiness, "and we can see scarring and hemorrhaging too close to your optic nerve to let us cut any further."

"I can see a little something," I said, "but nothing in front of me." What I saw was light and shadow coming through what seemed like the outer ring of a dart board, and even that was hazy, as if I were in a smoky room. "Won't it improve?"

"I'm sorry, no." He had a quiet, sincere voice, and I sympathized with him for what he had to tell me. "The peripheral vision you have in your left eye is all you will ever have."

That's it? I asked myself, but didn't say aloud. I didn't want the doctor to feel worse than he already did. But if this was all I was going to get, it wasn't much.

Still, my right eye works, I thought, desperate for a silver lining. My spider and amoeba pals remained in that eye, but I'd become expert at maneuvering my head to see around them. I vowed to become even more adept, now that I could hold my head up again.

Finally he asked if I had any more questions.

"No," I said, surprising us both.

———

Once I was home, we resumed our routine of Friday drives to Chicago, now for post-op exams on my left eye and laser treatments on the right. I loved being back in our apartment again, but day-to-day life was no easier than before the surgery.

When I returned to work after the operations, my boss, who understandably had her own struggle with my condition, made an appointment for me to go to the university's Rehab Center. "Maybe there's something there for people in your situation," she said. *People in my situation?* Just what was my situation, I wondered. I couldn't really see but I wasn't blind. As far as I was concerned, I didn't need any services the Rehab Center had to offer.

My boss had been great about granting time off and working

around my absences, but she wasn't particularly sensitive about what I was going through at the office. Co-workers, however, were very supportive, especially after that first unsuccessful surgery. When it came time to prepare for the national convention we went to each year, a colleague agreed to share a hotel room and help me negotiate any elevators or stairs that might be dangerous. I was very grateful. I always looked forward to the conventions and didn't want to miss this one.

One morning my co-workers and I were discussing plans for this meeting when the boss came out and called me into her office. Rubbing the back of my left hand along her door as a guide, I entered and was told to take a seat.

"I've decided you can't go to the conference, Beth," she said. She didn't want me to embarrass the office.

I was stunned. Had I looked that strange and awkward this whole time? Why had no one else ever told me? Was she the only one with enough courage or authority to speak up?

I skipped the conference. And made an appointment at the Rehab Center.

Long before it was a matter of law, the University of Illinois had earned a reputation for accommodating disabled students. A department and a building are dedicated to this effort; for decades buses with wheelchair lifts have ferried students to and from classes and the Center for Rehabilitation Education.

Mike dropped me off and I used my walking stick to find my way clumsily to the office of Janet Floyd, Director of Services for the Sensory Impaired. Luckily, she was a lot less formal than her title suggested.

"Have you ordered a white cane yet?"

I suppose I shouldn't have been surprised at the question.

"I won't need one."

She nodded an OK. "How have you been getting to work?"

"Sometimes I get a ride from my husband, sometimes I walk."

"Oh, that's great. You must live close to campus."

"Yeah," I said, a bit less defensive now. She must have been worried that I was still driving. "We're only five blocks from my office. I use this stick," I said, pointing. "Helps with curbs."

"If that's working for you, great." Janet was upbeat and personable. "If you ever feel the need to take a bus, you are eligible to use the Rehab Center's bus to get around campus."

"Thanks."

"We also have a couple of computers here that use speech synthesis."

My expression must have told her I didn't know what she was talking about. She laughed.

"They talk—they tell you what you're typing as you type."

"Oh, I don't need anything like that," I answered, feeling my defensive streak rising again. "I use regular computers." I explained that our office had just started using personal computers a year earlier, in 1984. "I can still work with the word-processing program if I

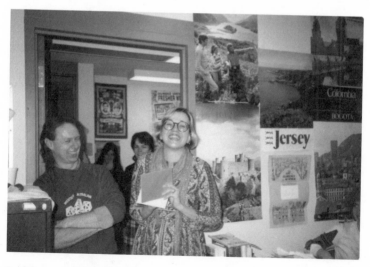

I celebrate my birthday with co-workers at the University of Illinois, 1984.

turn my office lights off and lean toward the screen." It had taken me a while to learn word processing; I sure didn't want to tackle speech synthesis.

"Wonderful," she said, settling me down again.

I liked Janet. She accepted my answers without getting superior. None of this I-know-what-you-need-more-than-you-do stuff. She just described the available services and invited me to call her whenever I needed anything.

Once this was over, we started talking about more interesting things. Janet wasn't much older than I was, and we found ourselves trading stories about our jobs, our families, where we'd gone to school. Janet was battling Hodgkin's disease and was in remission. I told her about life with diabetes. The hour flew by. Walking out, I thought about how gratifying it was to meet someone with such a store of positive energy, a woman who had ambitions despite her cancer. But her question about the white cane, and the image of myself actually using one, continued to gnaw at me.

Neither Janet nor my boss could have known what was going to happen next, of course, but a week later they both seemed prescient.

Getting ready for work, I bent to tie my shoes. That one simple act. It happened much as it had with my other eye, as if a black window shade were being drawn.

This time I had no good eye left.

I could still see my way to the phone, so I calmly called the doctor's office in Chicago. Then I called my own office to say I wouldn't be coming in. Next I found my way to our bookshelves and located my photo albums. As the last bit of light in my right eye faded, I pored over them, memorizing everyone, everything. I tried not to cry, knowing it would cloud what little I could see. But finally I couldn't hold back.

Mike had already left for work. He always called once he arrived, and when he did, I tried to pull myself together and give him the news. He said he'd come right home. I asked him not to, wanting, I guess, to be alone and mourn. The doctor's office eventually returned my call, and the very next day we scheduled surgery for my right eye. Only two months earlier they had operated on the left one.

I was in recovery when Mike was told that there had been some trouble in the operating room. The laser machine had acted up, and the procedure had taken six hours, much longer than anticipated.

My left eye was already blind, and now, after this second surgery, my right eye was patched. No one had to scold me about keeping my head down this time. Though I'd been assured that the failure of my last surgery had nothing to do with rolling my head in the night, this time I was determined to leave no room for doubt. In my conscious daytime hours I reminded myself there was no reward to picking up my head—it wouldn't help me see anything. At night I fought off sleep, fearing I'd fall into a REM stage and forget where my head belonged. Day and night I resisted the constant urge to stretch my neck.

"Tell them not to visit," I instructed Mike again. This time everyone, aside from faraway friends in Champaign, knew better. It was surprising just how much the sounds of old familiar voices could bring cheer to a crummy hospital room.

My mom visited after this second surgery. After seeing her kids off to school, my sister Cheryl had picked her up, battled the traffic, braved the scary neighborhoods, and arrived early enough to spend a few hours with me. I was flattered, but bothered by the sadness and worry in my mom's voice. She seemed not to share my confidence that this surgery would succeed.

A day after that visit, the resident interrupted my morning exam and called in the specialist. Another blood vessel had burst in my right eye.

"We can operate again," the doctor told me, "or we can try something that won't require general anesthesia."

It was a weekday morning; Mike was working in Champaign and unavailable. I hated making this kind of decision alone, but I thought about it for all of a few seconds. Recalling the recoveries from the general anesthesia, I chose the outpatient procedure. It was scheduled for that afternoon.

An eyedrop baptism started immediately and continued throughout the morning. Some of the drops dilated my eye; others were supposed to numb it. Shortly after lunch my face was scrubbed. The surgeon and one of the residents wheeled me to outpatient surgery.

I am coldly suspicious of people's stories about childbearing, or passing kidney stones. If you can talk about it, it must not have been that bad.

So let me just say this: A long needle was inserted into my eyeball to suck out the bloody matter. Then it was used to inject new saline solution. And the topical anesthetic, well . . . not enough, not enough. When they returned me to my room I asked them to draw the curtains around my bed. I lay in a fetal position for hours, my head, of course, turned down, rimmed by the hemorrhoid doughnut.

Other operations and procedures followed, or so Mike tells me. To this day I simply can't or won't remember anything beyond that needle.

———

I was given the option of leaving the hospital early, on the condition that I keep my head down and return two or three times a week for checkups. I jumped at the chance.

Because my sister Cheryl has three kids, she had a *big* car with a *big* back seat. Though it might have seemed frivolous, she agreed to drive me down all the way to Champaign, just to be home, even if it was only for two days. I was able to lie face down for the whole trip. I couldn't hold up my end of the conversation, but Cheryl didn't complain.

I spent two days at home with Mike, two nights in my own bed. Then Cheryl and I headed back to Chicago for another doctor visit.

My oldest sister, Bobbie, lived in Downers Grove, a suburb about a half-hour from the Eye and Ear Infirmary, and she was happy to have me stay with her during my recovery. A cushioned redwood lounge chair was dragged into the house so I could lay with my head hanging over the edge. On nicer days we'd wheel the chair back outside, affording me one of life's simple pleasures: lying in the sunshine.

It was nice having family visit me at Bobbie's; I didn't feel obliged to entertain them as I might have at the hospital. I caught up with

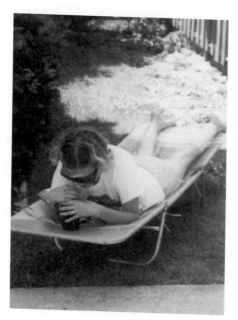

I had to remain facing down at all times following eye surgery, 1985.

Champaign friends by phone, rather than relying solely on Mike's weekly reports.

In fact, I got more help from my relatives at Bobbie's than I received from the nursing staff at the hospital. For example, the nurses often forgot that I needed an insulin shot before I could eat, so my hospital breakfasts usually grew cold. Not at Bobbie's. Like me, Bobbie is a Type I diabetic. She knew how to draw up insulin and always had a shot ready when I needed it.

Bobbie and Cheryl and another sister, Marilee, took turns as chauffeur and sighted guide when I visited the Eye and Ear Infirmary. Mike came up on weekends, and at the end of July he made arrangements to accompany me to my Monday appointment.

There was one piece of good news that day: the air bubble had finally dissipated, permitting the doctor to view the inside of my eye. The bad news was what he saw.

"I'm afraid there's nothing else we can do," he said in a tone that I recognized from his final report on my left eye.

All I could think to ask was, "Can I lift my head now?"

He said I could. Thankful for at least that, I raised my head for the first time in over a month. I was struck by a sudden feeling of freedom and relief: no more lasers, no more operations, no more weekly visits to Chicago, no more worrying whether or not this all was going to work.

I swiveled my head as if to look around. I saw nothing.

Mike talked to the doctor, asking sensible questions, I suppose. Turning toward their voices, I asked if this was really it. Had we exhausted every possibility?

"I'm a religious man," the doctor answered, "and in the religion I follow we believe in miracles. I believe God has cured all sorts of ailments. This could happen with you, but there's nothing else I can do for you medically."

We stood to leave. I reached out for his hand. He clasped mine with both of his, and I thanked him for all he had done. He was shaking. I felt sorry for him; I would have liked to tell him we were going to be all right.

The White Sox were in town that day. Going to a ball game after learning I'd be blind for the rest of my life was probably a strange thing to do, but it beat heading home and sitting on our pitiful second-hand couch and wondering where to turn next.

The team was having a rotten year. There were maybe eight thousand people in the stands, Floyd Banister pitched, and the Sox lost. But it was strangely pleasant, sitting next to Mike with my head up, not giving a thought to eyes or surgery. We each had a bratwurst and a beer. Between bites and gulps and giving me play-by-play, Mike bantered with other fans, cursing the underachievers on the team. I laughed at Nancy Faust, the Sox organist—she's famous for picking songs that allude to players' names. Mike marveled at the endurance of Carlton Fisk, and we both wondered aloud why it was that every time we attended a game, that bum Banister was pitching.

The three-hour ride home was quiet. Once back in Urbana, we found ourselves sitting on our miserable couch, as we'd feared, holding hands and wondering how we'd cope. Our only decision that night was to go to sleep. Our bed felt wonderful. I was home for good. Despite everything, a powerful relief came over me, a sense of security—such a change from how I'd felt during those months in my hospital bed.

And I realized right away that sight isn't needed under the covers.

1   My Two Companions

I was seven years old in 1966, when I was diagnosed with juvenile diabetes. My lasting memories of that period have mainly to do with urine: constantly going to the bathroom, wetting myself every night and almost every day. Although I went to Girl Scout day camp that summer, my recollections do not involve making a pair of beaded moccasins or swimming or learning clever campfire songs. All I remember is that the camp had outhouses, smelly outhouses.

My situation worsened until I rarely managed the entire bus ride home from camp without an "accident." I sat in the back, hoping no one would notice. The bus dropped us off at our elementary school, and from there I'd hurry home to clean up. One day a friend of my sister Cheryl decided to surprise me by picking me up in his Corvette. How I would have loved that ordinarily, the spectacle of riding in his convertible! Instead I was horrified. I didn't dream of telling him about my soiled outfit, and I was scared to death I'd wreck his car seat. All the way home I did my best to levitate.

My pee problem went on and on—I remember some suggestion that my incontinence might be "emotional." But later that summer our family joined Aunt Arjean, Uncle Ray, and cousin Randy, who was a juvenile diabetic, on a drive to visit some older relatives at their Wisconsin cabin. In our first hundred-mile stretch Uncle Ray had to pull the car over four times to let me squat in roadside cornfields. Aunt Arjean became suspicious about my symptoms. When we arrived at the cabin, she used one of my cousin's urine test strips to check me. The visit was cut short, and next thing I knew, I was in the hospital.

Diabetes is an absolutely diabolical disease. With as many as twenty-four thousand new cases of blindness caused by diabetes each year, it's the leading cause of blindness in adults. Diabetes accounts for 40 percent of new dialysis and kidney transplant patients—about thirty thousand per year—and is therefore the leading cause of kidney failure in adults as well. It leads to circulatory problems that can cause nerves in the fingers, hands, toes and feet to go numb, or, sometimes, to scream out in pain. Poor circulation is also why diabetes is a leading cause of impotence in males.

Low blood sugars can cause a diabetic to become unresponsive and pass out; high blood sugars can fill the vascular system with toxic ketones and acid, causing diabetic coma. Wounds heal slower in diabetics, sometimes leading to gangrene. Diabetes is the most frequent cause of non-traumatic lower limb amputation.

Diabetes hastens cardiovascular disease. A middle-aged person with diabetes is two to four times more likely to have a stroke than is a non-diabetic.

In short, diabetes effectively compromises and shortens millions of lives.

Diabetes is a confusing and misunderstood disease, due in no small part to all the different names and terminology used to describe it. Take juvenile diabetes, which is also known as Type I, or insulin-dependent diabetes. Somewhere along the line the term "juvenile" stuck, because Type I diabetes most often develops in kids. Yet it's not uncommon for adults to develop it. (My sister Bobbie has "juvenile" diabetes, even though she was diagnosed in her late twenties.)

In juvenile or Type I diabetes the pancreas simply shuts down. More precisely, the cells that produce insulin, cells that happen to reside in the pancreas, stop functioning. Insulin is a hormone that allows the body to metabolize sugars. Without it, sugars (and starches that are converted to sugars) cannot be processed, and so pass right through the system. That's why I had to pee so much back when I was seven—what I drank and ate ran straight through me. It's also why I was so skinny. Without insulin, diabetics effectively starve to death, unable to take nutritional value from food. That was the fate of Type I diabetics until scientists learned that insulin injections could provide some approximation of normal pancreatic function.

Type I diabetes is a matter of heredity, not behavior. Type I diabetics seem to be born with a trait that incapacitates insulin-producing cells. It runs in families (my cousin, my sister, and me). Many theories have been suggested to explain how and why this happens. The most intriguing these days is that something causes the immune system suddenly to misidentify the insulin-producing cells as intruders. The body then attacks and destroys these cells, just as it might attack a transplanted organ.

Research on Type I diabetes is being conducted on many fronts. On the genetic side, scientists are trying to pinpoint the trait that causes the body to turn on itself. There are also ongoing trials in which children with a family history of the disease are monitored and given anti-rejection drugs to head off its onset.

For thirty-five years now, doctors have been performing pancreas transplants—or, more commonly, kidney-pancreas transplants. The kidney is added to the equation because diabetes is particularly destructive to parts of the body, such as the eyes or kidneys, that rely on very small blood vessels. When successful, the transplants restore the recipients' ability to produce insulin. But they are major operations. The anti-rejection drugs carry their own well-known difficulties, and organs are in short supply. Another approach, one I find the most promising, involves transplanting only the insulin-producing cells. Problems remain, but recent trials have produced good results, so there's reason for Type I's to be optimistic.

In Type II (also known as adult onset) diabetes, the insulin-producing cells are overwhelmed, rather than destroyed. Typically some condition or combination of conditions—obesity or age—brings it on. The insulin-producing cells continue to function, but they can't keep up. Type II diabetics can often "cure" themselves by losing enough weight to bring their demand for insulin in balance with their ability to produce it. Of course, losing weight is easier said than done, and often Type II diabetics can't manage it. They (and Type II diabetics who are compromised for other medical reasons) may require oral medication or insulin injections to control the disease.

The dirty little secret among diabetics is that we Type I's resent Type II's: We think they give us all a bad name. This is less their fault than a symptom of how frightening is the prospect of serious illness. Because people want to believe the afflicted are to blame, they focus on avoidable behaviors. "Well, he smoked," they think when a friend gets cancer, or "She was a couch potato," when a co-worker experiences heart trouble. When people find out I'm diabetic, they often boast to me about not letting their children (or sometimes themselves) eat sweets. Diabetes runs in the family, they explain, so they have to be careful. I wonder whether they know the difference between Type I and Type II, or which one runs in their family. I assume they think I stuffed myself with ice cream and cookies as a child, or, worse yet, that my beloved mom—I affectionately call her by her first name, Flo—let her seven kids gorge on sweets. It makes me mad.

But I can't claim we Type I's are angels when it comes to casting blame. "All those Type II's need to do is lose weight," we tell ourselves. We would kill for that option. And we despise the overweight Type II's for contributing to the supremely aggravating myth that our disease is somehow traceable to eating too many sweets. Insofar as M&Ms and Twinkies contribute to a weight problem, yes, they could lead to Type II diabetes. But Type I's are the *righteous* diabetics. For us, *it's heredity, dammit!*

So don't confuse the two diseases. It's serious business—research dollars and potential breakthroughs hang in the balance. I can't help believing we'd all be better served if there were separate names for these very different diseases.

While Type I's still await an outright cure, there has been important incremental progress in how the disease is managed. Management is commonly thought to be a matter of avoiding high blood sugars. That's true, as far as it goes, but you can take too much insulin and drive blood sugars dangerously low. The Holy Grail of sugar levels is 100 milligrams per deciliter (mg/dL). Test a non-diabetic's blood at any given time and the reading will be around 100. Diabetics always shoot for that norm. Higher levels create conditions where the extra sugar in the bloodstream can cause complications: kidney malfunctions, gangrene, or blindness.

When is blood sugar too low? That varies from person to person. There's a stage, whether at 70 or 50 mg/dL, where you feel drunk. You get giddy, or maybe you get nasty. If someone asks if you're all right, you'll swear that you're fine, but your judgment is off. Below this level, things can become very problematic. You can simply black out. This could happen when you're driving. Even the diabetic under good control is never far from hazards of low sugars.

Diabetes management is also made difficult by the complex interplay of diet and exercise. The human body—a healthy one—ingeniously monitors itself, constantly altering the amount of insulin it produces to suit the situation. During and after a big meal, it pumps out insulin. During exercise or between meals, production slows. The body adjusts for illness, pregnancy, adolescence, stress, and other conditions. Remember that 100 mg/dL? The average non-diabetic, despite these variables, will still test out to about 100, whereas even a religiously diligent diabetic can spike to 300 or 400 with the onset of the flu. Over time, too many high numbers can result in horrendous diabetic complications.

When I was diagnosed in 1966, I spent two weeks in the hospital. Doctors armed my mom with urine test strips, syringes, insulin vials, and menu sheets to use after my release. I took one shot a day at home. My mother and I would conduct urine tests, record the results, and show them to my doctor at my semi-annual appointments. Based on those tests, he might adjust my daily insulin and/or suggest a change in diet.

Today, a newly-diagnosed seven-year-old Type I diabetic might still be admitted to the hospital, but only for a day or so. She and her parents would go home with an electronic blood glucose monitor that, while still requiring finger pricks, makes glucose testing convenient enough to perform several times daily. She might use two kinds of insulin, one long acting, the other short. She'd likely take three to six shots a day, and—working with her doctor or nurse practitioner—her parents could adjust her insulin levels on a weekly, daily, or even shot-to-shot basis, depending on test results. She might even be given an insulin pump, a little box attached to a tiny tube that connects to her body through a needle under her skin. Worn under clothing or on a belt, the pump continually delivers a base level of insulin and allows her to pump more insulin at meals by pushing a button.

The net effect for the girl diagnosed today is a smoother tightrope walk, a narrower range of blood sugars on a daily basis. A bigger hassle for her in the short run, but over the long haul she'll be much, much less likely to suffer diabetic complications such as blindness.

Yet, fundamentally, today's seven-year-old faces the same reality I confronted in the 1960s. She and her parents have more tools, but she is still insulin dependent; if anything, all the new technologies mean that insulin dependence will disrupt her day-to-day life even more than it did mine. She'll have to come to terms with this unwanted companion, as I did.

Or didn't.

When I was seven, my two-week hospital stay mainly meant gifts and extra attention, and the promise that, if I took my shot every day, I wouldn't wet my pants anymore. The special attention continued when I returned home.

"Don't eat that! That's for Beth!"

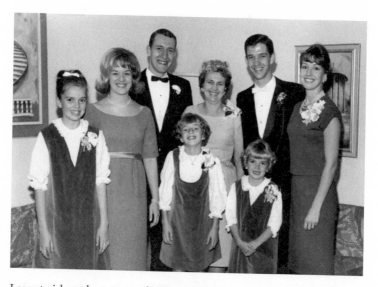

Lowest girl on the totem pole, surrounded by my six siblings and Flo, at Doug's wedding, 1964. From left: Marilee, Cheryl, Ron, Beverle, Flo, Doug, Beth, and Bobbie.

"You'll have to wait. Beth needs to eat first."

These admonitions to my siblings became typical in our house. My notoriety was precious in a family where there were seven kids and a widowed mom working full time.

For a long while after my hospital discharge I slept with Flo to help her detect any nighttime low blood sugar attacks. I'd wake up to the smell of a special breakfast cooking just for me, then hear a *click, click, click.* It was her wedding ring striking the glass as she rolled the insulin vial gently between her hands. Nurses had instructed her to mix up the insulin before using it, but not to shake the bottles too much. "If you get bubbles in there, they'll end up in the syringe," they warned. Morning injections from Flo became as routine as brushing my teeth. A needle prick was a small price to pay for all that one-on-one attention each morning before she left for work.

Flo had served as den mother for my Boy Scout brothers long before I was born. She hadn't done anything like that since, never a Scout leader or even a room mother for any of my sisters. But now, having just turned fifty, she became a co-leader of my troop. *How else would Beth be able to go on campouts,* she reasoned.

The two of us were parked near a campfire the one time I remember complaining to her about diabetes. "I want hot chocolate!" I was crying, and she scooted over in the front seat of the car to hug me. Somehow from the one-syllable words she uttered—"aw" and "Beth" and "oh"—I knew I wasn't wrong to feel sad.

Staying sad, however, would have been wrong by Flo's reckoning. Once I calmed down, she took a handkerchief out of her purse, wet it with her tongue, and cleaned off my face. We went to the campfire. I sang songs while the other girls drank hot chocolate and ate s'mores.

At school I was the only kid allowed to have candy in my desk, to remedy low blood sugar attacks. The school nurse kept orange juice in the refrigerator, my name printed with Magic Marker over the label. She kept urine strips there for me, too, although the container collected dust. I knew how to test my urine, knew I was *supposed* to do it four times a day, but rarely bothered. "It's gross," I thought, "and I feel fine, so why bother?"

I was nine years old before I gave myself an injection. For two years I'd been practicing with used syringes, drawing water out of a cup and sticking the needle into an orange, just to get the feel of it. I'd take my dolls out and give them shots, too. My eleven-year-old sister Beverle, closest to me in age and the one I fought with the most, sometimes joined me at the kitchen table during practice sessions. Playing with syringes remains one of the few things I remember the two of us enjoying together as children.

My mom never pressured me to take my own shot, but eventually I decided I wanted to. In fourth grade, when I was invited to my first slumber party, I knew I wouldn't be able to go unless I could

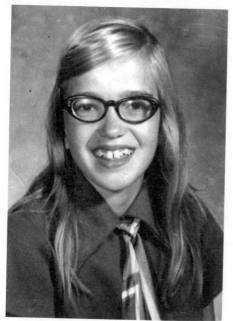

By 1970 I was a typically glamorous seventh grader—and I was administering my own insulin shots.

inject myself in the morning. A week before the party, I could draw the insulin into the syringe, pinch up some skin on my thigh and rub it with an alcohol patch. I could bring the needle within inches of my leg and tighten my eyes shut. But I couldn't muster the nerve to stick that needle into my own leg.

Nine was too young for an overnight party anyway, my mom said, making me all the more determined.

Two days before the party, I finally did it. "Good girl!" my mom exclaimed, seeing me stick the needle in my thigh and push the plunger down. After watching me take the needle out again, she gave me a quick hug and ran to the kitchen to check on my poached eggs.

The delight gained from knowing I'd be sleeping over with friends that weekend far exceeded any satisfaction I might have derived from finally giving myself the shot.

But then I got to the slumber party. The girls crowded around me when it was time for my injection. "That's neat!" they said as they watched me draw insulin from a vial. A chorus of oohs, ahs and ouches came out when I stuck the needle in my thigh; when I withdrew it, the birthday girl said *Wow, that was really brave.* I bent the needle back and forth to break it off, then made the other girls jealous by awarding the used syringe to the birthday girl. She told me later that it was her favorite gift.

By the time I was eleven or twelve my diabetes was less of a novelty at home, and in junior high everyone was much too concerned with their own bodies to care much about me and my shots. The disease pretty much left me alone until high school. I was a late bloomer, and the changes of adolescence wrought havoc with my body chemistry. Add all the normal stuff like wanting to fit in and you have a recipe for disaster.

In 1972, at the beginning of my freshman year, I was admitted to the hospital twice, both times close to coma. In the first episode, I could still talk when we arrived at the emergency room. In the second one, Flo found me in a heap on the basement floor and dragged me, a hundred pounds of dead weight, out the back door and into the car. During that second hospitalization, my doctor, exercising his version of bedside manner, declared that I wouldn't live past age thirty. Maybe he said it to scare me into taking better care of myself—test my urine more often, stick to my diet—I don't know. But, like lots of kids my age I suppose, I took him strictly at his word.

The effect of his prediction wasn't necessarily the one he intended. True, I worked harder at staying healthy, but this had to do with wanting to steer clear of the hospital. What his Nostradamus routine did was spark a sense of urgency: I wanted to squeeze in a full life before I turned thirty.

From then on I said yes to almost any opportunity for adventure that came my way. Most things I did were far from reckless: joining the high school band, learning to tap dance for the spring musical, running for student council, writing for the school newspaper. But I played with the dark side, too: going to rock concerts, smoking dope, ignoring Flo's curfews, finding bars in seedy neighborhoods that served underage drinkers, And, worst of all, eating ice cream.

My fall from diabetic grace began when a friend from band started working at Baskin-Robbins. She got another friend a job, then another friend, and so on. Soon the ice cream place became our hangout.

"Sugar-free" was not one of the thirty-one options back then, so for countless visits I stood aside and ate nothing while everyone else ordered. Then one time I tried a bite of a friend's cone, and guess what? I didn't die. This was proof enough for a fifteen-year-old: Ice cream must be OK for diabetics. I started out with single cones, then doubles. Eventually I was eating pints at a sitting.

Today, one could theoretically take a shot of fast-acting insulin to counteract the sugar and other calories in the ice cream. Back then, such insulin didn't exist. The two shots I took each day were long-acting insulins, far too slow and weak to handle the sugar jolt from pints of Pralines and Cream and Chocolate Mint Chip. For me, a teenage diabetic, ice cream was as risky as heroin.

I landed in the hospital again when I was sixteen, and it cured me of my habit. The blip on my popularity chart peaked off the screen when I returned to high school after being discharged. It was cool to know someone who had almost been in a coma.

Dating someone like that, however, was not so cool. I suppose I was lucky that sex never came up during my "Say yes to everything" days. Gangly and flat-chested, I was everyone's pal, nobody's temptress.

In my senior year I started ditching school once a week. The ditch days weren't planned ahead of time. A group of us would regularly huddle before first period to assess our assignments and test schedules, deciding whether it might be a good day to catch a commuter train to Chicago. Back then we thought it was a coincidence that everyone in this group had only one parent at home. Of course, now I realize that was the only way we could pull this off. Each of us got home from school before our single working parent got home from work, so we could snatch any unexcused absence reports from the mailbox.

In Chicago we'd walk to Michigan Avenue looking for nice restaurants—the fancier the restaurant, the less likely we'd be asked for identification when liquor was ordered. We'd sip wine with lunch, sure that no one suspected we were suburban high school kids.

I paid for these Chicago outings with tips from my waitress job. My budget didn't allow traveling, but that didn't keep me away from the airport. On nights when friends and I got antsy, we'd drive to the international terminal at O'Hare. A glassed-in balcony gave us a bird's-eye view of foreigners as they passed through customs. I learned to check information screens for news of Arab or African airline arrivals, as those travelers wore the most interesting clothes. Best of all was when officials asked for suitcases to be opened. Seeing all those personal belongings laid out in front of us was like going to a cultural museum.

—— ——

I became more resourceful—and had more resources—once I graduated from high school and started at the University of Illinois. I flew by myself for the first time in 1979, using Social Security benefits (as a survivor of my deceased father) and scholarships to pay for an internship in Washington, D.C. Later I employed a similar formula to cover my last semester of college in Salzburg, Austria, on a study abroad program that provided housing with an Austrian family. I loved leaving my world and dropping into someone else's, getting to know them, their perspectives, the little details that made their daily routines different from mine.

I received my bachelor's degree in 1980, but my wanderlust continued. To fund my habit I waitressed or found other part-time work at each stop, saving until I had enough for a ticket to the next destination.

I'd filled out some since high school, my braces were off now, and my wire-rimmed glasses were replaced by contact lenses. More confident about my looks, I was having the occasional romantic fling, but nothing serious. Which suited me fine; I wanted to keep moving. And getting serious would've required some heavy discussions about syringes and blood tests.

Most of the time I kept my diabetes to myself—I wasn't ashamed of it, but I never wanted it to be the most memorable thing about me. Having a fling was tricky, though. One of the joys of new love is its spontaneity: deciding at the last minute to stop for a bite to eat, staying up late, going for bike rides, the very kinds of irregularities that are a diabetic's nightmare. Early on in relationships, I didn't want boys to see my syringes or watch me weirding out during an attack of low blood sugar. I tried to be prepared for the unexpected

food stop or spur-of-the-moment walk together. Unlike the genet-
ically derived insulin used today, insulin back then was formulated
from beef and pork and had to be constantly refrigerated. I couldn't
carry it with me. If we stopped for an unplanned meal, I pretended
I wasn't hungry and ordered only a diet soft drink. This could bother
my date—it could seem like I was holding back. But in those days I
preferred taking that chance over bringing up all the diabetic stuff.

Surprise walks and bike rides presented the risk of low-blood-
sugar episodes. The amount of insulin I take in the morning depends
to a large degree on how much physical activity I expect that day. If
I know I'm swimming laps, I take less. If I think I won't be exercising at all, I take more. To counteract low blood sugars that might
arise, I am supposed to carry snacks with me. Back then, the last
thing I wanted was for a new boyfriend to see me in a semi-drunk-
en hypoglycemic state. Nor did I want him to see me scarfing candy before every bit of exercise. And, trivial as it sounds now, I
couldn't be bothered with transferring cookies, raisins, and crack-
ers from one pair of jeans to the next, from my shorts to my skirts.
I wanted to be spontaneous and unencumbered. Stupid, I know—
but in my late teens and early twenties, I *was* stupid. Eventually I
compromised and carried candies small enough to slip into my
mouth, unnoticed, before any strenuous activity.

To tackle the last-minute-bite-to-eat problem, I contrived to
make a quick stop at home first. Though puzzled, guys would always
oblige. I slipped my insulin out of the refrigerator and stole into the
bathroom. I think some guys wondered if I refrigerated my tampons
for thrills. They never asked—I think they were afraid to.

So I fashioned my Rube Goldberg solutions to the problems of
early romance. Diabetes-wise, at least. There were the more average
problems, like figuring out whether you actually had anything in
common. On the occasions when things went well, there were sec-
ond-stage challenges. What if we spend the night—do I have my
insulin with me? If not, I needed to be up and out early so I could

go home, take my shot, and eat breakfast as usual. Even if I had syringes and insulin with me, I had to gauge whether I'd already taken enough or would need more. After all, sex could be strenuous—or not. "Is all this going to be worth it?" I'd wonder.

It did eventually dawn on me that if I was fond enough of a guy to sleep with him, I ought to be able to tell him the truth about myself. Funny, though: When I finally tried this approach and asked to leave an extra bottle of insulin and some syringes in his refrigerator, the passion died.

One of my trips back then was to Philadelphia, to see a friend I'd met during my Washington internship. It typified the travel I did in those days, on a whim, on a shoestring. I'd spotted an odd ride-sharing ad in the campus newspaper: a student pilot wanted to accrue hours with an instructor in a certain plane; he was trying to scare up four passengers to help with the cost of renting it. I called and learned I could fly round-trip for well under a hundred bucks. "What's the catch?" I asked, as if flying with a novice weren't enough.

He said we'd have an overnight layover in Washington.

I told him I'd get back to him.

In my address book I found Michael Knezovich's work number. Mike and I had met in a journalism class a couple of years earlier—in fact, he's the one who'd told me about the internship program and encouraged me to try for it.

Apart from that, I'd had a crush on him ever since I'd first watched him stroll into class. He wore faded blue jeans, an oxford shirt with the sleeves turned up a couple of times. His shoulders and chest seemed huge compared to his narrow waist, small butt and strong, trim legs. His shirt was unbuttoned just far enough to show a hairy chest, and he had beautiful shoulder-length, reddish-brown hair, a full beard and mustache. Oh my. The layover in Washington didn't seem like such a bad idea.

We hadn't spoken since college, though—I didn't even know if he was still in D.C. But no one's ever accused me of bashfulness.

Mike answered the phone himself. I may have remembered him vividly, but it took him a moment to place me. When he did, he seemed pleased, or at least entertained by my chutzpah, and agreed to pick me up at the University of Maryland airport and put me up for the night.

He met me in his tiny yellow Ford Fiesta, right on time. Did I want to do a little sightseeing? Sure, I said. We headed to Old Town Alexandria and ended up in an Irish bar, drinking beers and trading tales. A researcher and writer for a consumer magazine, Mike loved his job but not his life in Washington. He had a case of the post-college blues and so was happy to hear me gab about life in Champaign-Urbana and my travel exploits. We had a great time.

He drove us to the place he was house-sitting and showed me my room. I have to admit I was hoping for a proposition that night. No luck. Next morning we had breakfast and he returned me to the airport. We hugged goodbye, and I climbed into the little plane. I saw Mike waiting for us to become airborne.

The pilot started down the runway, which suddenly became hugely bumpy. I looked outside. We were no longer on pavement. The flight instructor confirmed this, placidly informing us that we'd all need to help lift the plane back onto the tarmac.

Mike reached us in no time. He seemed both concerned and angry. He offered to help and was assigned a position. Then it was "One, two, *three*!" and we hefted the craft.

To this day I love to tease Mike with that story. Without fail he'll reply, "I should have known right then that you'd be a pain in the ass."

I saw Mike once more while he lived in Washington. It was 1981, and the friend I'd visited in Philadelphia had asked me to be in her wedding. Mike was my date. He took pains to leave work early on a Friday and join me at the rehearsal and dinner. Problem was, I'd given him the wrong time. He came bursting into the church, thinking he was late, but found it empty. He managed to keep his humor, and the two of us had a good time serving as bumpkin Midwesterners at a Philadelphia Main Line wedding. Except for a kiss or two, things remained platonic. I learned later I wasn't the problem. His last summer at school, Mike had fallen head over heels for someone who subsequently broke his heart. When I'd dropped in on his life, then later at the wedding, he still hadn't quite recovered.

I wrote him several times but put him out of my mind when I received no replies. Two years later, in 1983, he phoned out of the blue to say he'd quit his job and was visiting friends in Champaign. We made plans for a picnic lunch on the campus Quad.

Things had changed for both of us. Mike was over the college girlfriend. Moreover, he'd had the revelation that he just wasn't a Washingtonian or an East Coast guy in general. He'd quit his job and headed back to the Midwest, intent on settling in Chicago. Me? I'd gotten tired of doing cartwheels to keep my diabetic hassles out of view. I guess it was kind of like being a single mom: If a guy could deal with it, fine; if not, fine, too. I'd grown comfortable with the idea of being on my own.

So we brown-bagged it on the grass, neither of us burdened with expectations. I pulled out a Diet Pepsi, and Mike (who I'd learn has an absolute aversion to diet soda) asked, "Why do you drink that stuff?" It was a perfect entree, and I took it.

"I'm diabetic," I answered so nonchalantly I surprised myself.

"Oh," Mike answered. "I knew a kid in grade school who had diabetes. You take shots?"

"Three or four times a day."

He was actually kind of fascinated by it, asking questions until his curiosity was satisfied. We talked about our respective plans. With lunch over far too quickly, we made arrangements to go out that night. This time he did proposition me. Or maybe I propositioned him. Either way, he spent the night with me. And witnessed me testing my blood, taking my shots, and eating my oatmeal in the morning. He was unfazed.

He went back to Washington, retrieved his motorcycle and his belongings, and moved in with friends until he could find work and somewhere to live. From then on we spent virtually all our free time together. Mike found odd construction jobs, sandblasting buildings, digging trenches, until he settled into freelance technical writing for local companies.

Once I asked him why he hadn't pursued me while we were still in school. "I mean," I said, "how could you possibly have resisted me in my overalls?"

"God, those overalls!" he groaned. "You always looked like you'd just jumped out of bed and run to class."

"That's only because I had," I said. But then I pushed him a little more. He realized I'd had a crush on him.

"The thing was," Mike said kind of ruefully, "I was at the stage where someone approachable didn't measure up. It was like, you know, a simple case of 'Wouldn't want to be a member of any club that would accept me.' I was too busy pursuing women I had nothing in common with, the ones who were bound to break my heart."

By the time of our lunch on the Quad, I had settled down quite comfortably. I had a full-time position with the university, with benefits. I needed the health insurance to help pay for managing my disease: syringes, insulin, doctor visits and lab tests. (But that was just peanuts. I couldn't have known it then, but the health insurance that came with that job would keep us afloat later, when we would incur hundreds of thousands of dollars of medical bills.)

In 1983, my life as a diabetic was under fairly good control. In particular, I'd managed to acquire a blood glucose monitor. The monitors so commonplace now were new in the early 1980s, and expensive. Insurance covered neither the price of the machine nor, more important, the ongoing expense of the test strips. (Today, manufacturers often give their monitors away to market the strips, and many insurers cover the strips, at least partially.)

Not until my grandmother died in the early 1980s, leaving me a small windfall, could I afford a monitor. Armed with the new machine, I could manage my sugar levels better and began to feel confident I'd make a liar out of the doctor who'd forecast my demise within the coming decade. I had less confidence that I'd escape the long-term complications of the disease. I feared the damage already done. I might make it past thirty, but maybe not without kidney failure or losing a limb to gangrene. Or maybe he'd be proven right in one regard: I wouldn't *see* my thirtieth birthday, because by then I'd be blind.

I had also been told years earlier that diabetic women should not have babies, that pregnancy raises the chances of diabetic complications, and that most times the pregnancy ends in a stillbirth.

It was Mike's presence in my life that started shifting these thoughts to the forefront of my consciousness. I'd written off the prospect of having any lifelong companion other than diabetes, but Mike had changed all that. And I began to worry. He may have learned about syringes and insulin and glucose monitors, but I'd yet to tell him about the nasty things the disease could do to me.

I had fallen in love with the twin cities of Champaign-Urbana back in 1976, during my freshman year at the University of Illinois. It didn't matter that there was nowhere to hike or canoe, or that the campus was surrounded by (even included) corn and soybean fields. It seemed a vibrant place. I was caught up in the rush of thirty-five thousand students hustling from class to class. Now, working full-time, I was every bit as fond of it, though I'd started living the life of a townie.

When Mike and I were dating, I lived east of campus in a typical Urbana rental house, built in 1906 for a single family but converted more recently to an up-and-down duplex. I had the downstairs unit, kind of beat up on the inside (especially the kitchen, with its hodgepodge of aging appliances). Even so, it had character. Like other houses in the neighborhood, it had a front porch swing.

Champaign-Urbana may lack a striking natural beauty—it defines the word "flat," and the creek that trickles through it, more of a drainage ditch, is known as The Boneyard. But what the two towns have, especially Urbana, is trees. Huge, magnificent old maples and oaks with an unearthly gift for turning brilliant scarlet and sunset yellow. A few white clouds set against a deep blue sky on an autumn afternoon—we could watch them indefinitely from our vantage point on the porch swing.

And on a splendid September day in 1983, that's exactly what Mike and I did. Swinging back and forth, holding hands, we quietly soaked in the colors. Long after sunset, when we could no longer see even the brightest orange leaves, we finally went inside to cook dinner in my old kitchen.

Cleaning up later, drying dishes and handing them to Mike to put back into their dingy cupboards, probably the most unromantic moment of a memorable afternoon and evening, I suddenly knew I was in love. I was seized by an inexplicable mix of feelings, being completely at ease while at the same time being terribly excited, wanting to grab hold of him, to hug him fiercely and not let go.

So I did. Hold him, I mean. Mike either felt the same thing at the same time or at least recognized what was going on. Suddenly, in a burst, I found myself telling him everything—the likelihood of my never having children, the odds that I'd lose my kidney function, an appendage, my eyesight, my life.

Mike held my hand and listened. When I was finished, he asked a few questions, kissed me and said he thought it might be a good idea to go home and think for a couple of days. Given everything I'd dumped on him, I had to agree.

This talk of ours hadn't been about marriage or engagement or anything like that. But neither of us had ever had a long-term relationship; this seemed to be heading in that direction, and I wanted to make sure Mike understood what he might be in for. I already knew I loved him, and I wanted things to continue. But he needed to understand that if he kept things going, he'd be taking up me and my constant companion, diabetes.

Days went by with no word from Mike. Some women might have worried, but I was thankful; I wanted him to take as much time as he needed, and I was glad he apparently understood the gravity of what I told him.

Finally he called and offered to come over and make dinner. Before the cooking started, he sat at the kitchen table and said, "Well, I thought about what you said."

I feigned surprise. "You did?"

He looked up and saw me smiling. He grunted and then finally smiled at my little remark. But in an instant his tone became serious again.

Mike has always been able to express himself well—to me, at least—in important moments. He credits this talent to his vivid imagination. Most of his quiet time, he says, is spent thinking through different scenarios, analyzing, anticipating outcomes.

Sitting back in my chair, I tried to brace myself for what was coming. "The more I thought about it," he started, "I mean, I should leave now. That way, I can avoid all the messy stuff that might happen to you down the road."

My heart sunk, but I was stoic. "Of course you should," I said, standing up to turn around so he wouldn't see me cry.

"Sit down!" he barked, breaking out of his clinical tone. "I'm not done."

I sat.

"But then I figured, if I leave, the bad things could still happen to you," he said. "I just wouldn't be there."

He waited for me to look at him.

"And that would be worse. I would want to be there. I would need to be there."

So that, said Michael Knezovich, was that. I was crying. He came over, and after wiping my tears he pulled me up to hug me. "And besides, no one could take care of you like I can."

Two days before Christmas 1983, Mike gave me an engagement ring. It was my twenty-fifth birthday. The following summer we were married in my sister Bobbie's backyard. If that airplane veering off the runway in Maryland had been an omen of the bad things headed our way, our wedding day symbolized all the good. Bobbie's husband, Harry, a whiz of a gardener, had their backyard looking like something out of *Town & Country*. The skies were blue and the temperature and humidity were more typical of spring than of late July. Everyone we'd wanted to have with us had somehow made it from points around the country. My friend Colleen's father, a judge,

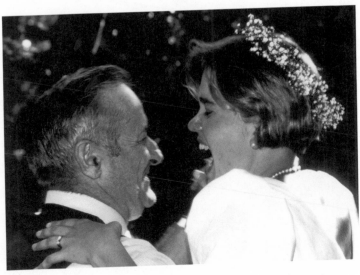

Mike's dad polkas with Mike's bride at the wedding reception, 1984.

married us in a private ceremony. Later, at the backyard gathering, Mike's friend Pick—his best pal from his Washington days—presided over our public exchange of the vows we'd written. Pick was raised a Virginia Baptist and studied drama in college. Colorful and animated, he played his role so well most people thought he was truly a minister.

Flo walked me down the aisle, and my friends Anne and Colleen served as bridesmaids. When it came time for a toast, the nieces and nephews served champagne. We'd hired a group of Mike's dad's buddies from the steel mill, Roland Kwasny and the Continentals, who moonlighted playing weddings and other functions. They were everything we could have hoped for. Behind bandstands monogrammed "RK," the ruffle-shirted, heavy-set machinists and bricklayers played everything from polkas to "Proud Mary." And Roland and the boys were good enough to let Pick—a versatile showman, indeed—sing a few numbers while my sister Beverle sat in on drums.

We ate and drank and danced until well after sundown. We told each other it was the best day of our lives.

2 | Braille Jail

"Rehabilitation" is a funny word. It brings to mind the Betty Ford Clinic, prisons and parole boards, shabby old houses. It means fixing something that's not right. I never liked thinking of myself that way, but rehabilitation was what I needed after the eye surgeon told me I would never see again.

My official rehabilitation began with a visit to the local office of the Illinois Department of Rehabilitation Services (DORS). It was in the summer of 1985; Mike and I had been married for a year. Mike had been doing freelance technical writing for different companies while I was in and out of the hospital that spring. Now he stopped looking for new projects because he wanted to be at home to help me. After driving me to the local DORS office, he led me to the waiting room, sat with me during the appointment, and filled out reams of paperwork so I could be assigned a caseworker. It turned out to be weeks before DORS took any action, so it was a good thing Mike was home.

With his help, I improvised. With painstaking care I learned to find the railing on the stairway out of our apartment, to locate our slot in the row of mailboxes at the foot of the stairs, to operate my Library of Congress tape recorder so I could hear books on tape. We rearranged furniture and kitchen utensils. We had no idea whether we were doing things by the blind rehab book, but we had no choice. And it was occasionally fun, coming up with little tricks and solving puzzles.

Typical of the problems I faced was putting toothpaste on my toothbrush. After a few mornings of seeing Crest plastered all over the bathroom sink (not to mention all over me), Mike suggested that I get my own tube and simply squirt it into my mouth. *Voilà.*

I often dropped things, and I soon learned that if I immediately froze and listened intently until the object stopped bouncing or rolling, I had a better chance of finding it. I "scanned" the floor with my hand, making progressively smaller arcs. Rubber bands became my friends. We put one on my hair conditioner so I wouldn't use it when I wanted shampoo, around the audio cassette on which Mike had recorded frequently used phone numbers, and around the aspirin bottle to distinguish it from other medicines. When rubber bands didn't work—say, to differentiate my apartment key from others—we'd use tape or stickers.

But there were scads of little tasks that I simply left to Mike. Pouring liquids, for example. I knew there must be a way for me to do so without spilling, but for the life of me I couldn't manage it. And cooking might as well have been calculus; I didn't know where to start, and the thought of my using sharp knives and a gas stove made Mike queasy.

In addition, I suffered from insomnia during those first months. Every time I awoke, I assumed it was time to get up. Mike suffered, too, because I'd nudge him and ask him what time it was. Eventually I tried instead to listen for the birds, but by the time I heard them, I was dead tired. Many mornings I ended up sleeping in.

━━   ━━

Each day when I slipped out of the covers, Mike made coffee and got my insulin ready. I still gave myself the injection, but we couldn't come up with a way for me to draw accurate doses. Over breakfast, we'd try to think of things to do that required neither money nor vision. The tradeoff for Mike's being at home with me was an extremely tight budget. We became embarrassingly addicted to TV game shows that we could both play, and we rarely missed *All My Children*.

Besides books on tape, my best daily diversion was my journal. Sometime during my hospitalizations a social worker suggested that I start writing down my experiences. A terrific idea, but as my sight worsened, it became impractical for me to write daily entries. The logical solution would have been for me to tape record them. But I thought then—and still think today—of "writing" as producing something on paper. Mike and I eventually came up with a convoluted scheme: I'd type the entry, then he'd read it onto tape so I could review what I'd written. (He'd sometimes chip in his own two cents' worth on the audio version.) Keeping that journal became a part of my daily routine.

I didn't get much exercise that summer, but I was usually exhausted by early evening. Concentrating on tiny details all day long took its toll. By six or seven o'clock my head was spinning with things like: *The denim-feeling garment is my dark blue jumper. The cotton shirt with two buttons on the shoulder is light-blue plaid; the one with buttons up the front is plain white. Brown shoes are on the floor on the left side of the closet; the closet is at the foot of the bed on the right side; the bed juts out from the wall near the bathroom door.*

To make things a little easier, I decided to purge the visually oriented stuff that got in my way and constantly reminded me of my sighted life. My books were first to go. I asked Mike which ones he wanted for himself. Feeling through his rejects, I could still identify some by touch. My *Children's Book of Literature* had a terribly loose binding; my *Riverside Shakespeare* had those almost gossamer pages; my *Le Petit Prince* was small and thin. At the last minute I kept a few, thinking I might parcel them out to special people over time. The rest went to a used bookstore. A few days later I collected all of my magazines and had them shipped to the doctor's office in Chicago. Now they could finally ditch that two-year-old copy of *Sports Illustrated*.

Next I tackled my clothes closet. I figured that if I got rid of half of what I owned, our closet wouldn't be so stuffed. There would be fewer textures, and I'd have an easier time identifying things. Shirts or skirts that felt too much alike were sent to nieces who wore my size.

My sheet music was more difficult. My sight-reading skills had been very good, and I'd collected scads of piano books, sheet music, even some hand-written stuff. I wanted to give it to someone who would appreciate it, someone who had admired and maybe even coveted my collection in the past. I stewed and stewed about this. You'd think I was giving away Liz Taylor's jewels. The sheet music wasn't worth much, but the act of giving it away had tremendous symbolic value to me. An old high-school friend finally came to mind, and we sent it to him.

Then there was the box of letters and cards from old friends, boyfriends, and family: the bits and pieces that constitute a loose chronicle of your life but that you seldom actually look at. Private, nostalgic things. I had no idea what I'd ever do with them; they were so personal that I wouldn't want someone else to see them in order to read them to me. In the end, I kept them. Kept my photo albums, too.

Mike and I got on remarkably well that summer, but we had our moments. Our biggest fight was over a hairbrush.

It was a typical weekday morning. Mike made coffee, poured some into my favorite cup, led me to a chair, and we planned our day. It was my turn to shower first.

I felt my way to the bathroom, checked the hook for my towel, turned on the hot water, waited for it to warm up, then added cold. Inside the shower, I wetted my hair and felt for the bottle without the rubber band: shampoo. Then the body soap, always kept directly under the nozzle so I wouldn't have to grope for it. When I finished, I flipped the shower lever to direct the water out the tub faucet before I turned off the water. That way, if I confused the handles, I wouldn't get scalded or frozen.

Back in my robe, I felt for the toothpaste—Mike's little suggestion made brushing tidy. Deodorant was also easy. I used roll-on; Mike used stick. And I could tell by the fragrance.

But putting on make-up? Forget it.

I turned the bathroom over to Mike, crossed the bedroom, and felt through the closet. It was hot, so I picked a sleeveless cotton dress. I thought it was light blue, but since I never wore anything with it, I hadn't bothered to memorize its color. I used my knee to feel around our bed to the dresser, where I kept my underwear in the top left drawer. I had stopped folding my panties, since feeling for them just unfolded them anyway. Thinking of the heat, I felt for a cotton pair. The tag should go on the left seam. Next, I searched the right-hand corner of the dresser for my hairbrush. In the old days, I could set my brush down wherever I'd used it last; now everything in our house had a place.

The brush wasn't there. I crouched and felt around the floor: nothing but dirt and dust. I stuck my hand under the dresser: only cobwebs. Perfume bottles and earring holders toppled as I groped the dresser's surface again. When I tried to set them upright, I knocked over things of Mike's. I quit searching. To this day, one of the most frustrating problems is trying to find something that I know is *right there.*

I touched my hair. It was already starting to dry, but Mike wasn't done in the shower. I didn't want to interrupt him—though I should have; it would have been kinder than to sit outside and fume.

What has he done with it? I asked myself. *And why would he have to use my brush anyway?* The more I thought about it, the angrier I became. *God, why does he have to take such a long shower?* I tried to pace but grew disoriented and paced myself right into a wall. I sat down again and tried to loosen the tangles with my fingers.

The shower finally quit running. I heard the door open.

"*Where's my brush?*"

My anger startled him; I could tell by the sound of his voice as he answered, "Right where it always is."

"*It is not!* Why don't you put stuff back when you use it? Don't you know how hard it is for me to find things when they're not where they are supposed to be?" I started to cry.

"Look at my hair. It's going to look stupid all day now." Mike tried to interrupt, but I wouldn't have it.

"You have to put everything back where it belongs! How do you expect me—"

Now Mike was angry. "Listen, I didn't use your goddamned brush, but even if I did, and even if I didn't put it back, I don't want you scolding me. I do my best, but I'm not a robot and I don't want to live like a goddamned Stepford wife! Besides, I'm better about putting things back than *you* are!"

I stopped crying. He was right: I was terrible about putting things where they belonged. But if he started leaving things out, how would I *ever* find them? And if I couldn't find things, how would I ever get *anything* done? What if I couldn't find my hairbrush one day after I had returned to work?

I took a deep breath. "Have you seen my brush?" I asked, almost in a whisper.

Mike took my hand, brought me to the dresser, and placed my palm on the hairbrush. It was about three inches closer to the center of the dresser than usual. It might as well have been a hundred yards away.

"Thank you," I said. I sat and brushed my hair.

——— ———

Weeks passed before my caseworker from the Department of Rehabilitation Services met with me and my boss. I expected to discuss talking computers, what we'd need to put one on my desk, when I could return to work, and so on. Instead, the caseworker talked about other tools and skills I would need before returning to the office. Braille was mentioned, as was orientation and mobility training. She explained that there was a residential school in Chicago that provided intensive training to newly blind adults.

"It's called the Illinois Visually Handicapped Institute," she continued. "I've sent clients there before."

"How long a program is it?" my boss asked.

"That really varies with each student. Three months is probably the minimum, but some students stay much longer."

"That sounds ideal," my boss said with a note of relief in her voice.

She seemed eager to make me someone else's problem. On the other hand, she also made it clear that, once I learned these skills, I could come back to work. I chose to focus on that. I'd be gone three months, work hard, and come back ready to reconstruct my life.

Mike and I filled out still more paperwork, and my caseworker reserved my spot at IVHI. We both dreaded my living away from home again, and we started calling IVHI "Braille Camp" to make light of the upcoming absence. It helped. The dread was gradually offset by high hopes and expectations.

In the fall Mike drove me to IVHI to begin my formal rehabilitation. It reminded me of being dropped off at my college dorm for the first time . . .

Except I wasn't going to school to learn new things so much as to learn how to do without old things.

Except now I was married and really didn't want to live away from home.

Except now I was blind.

— —

A volunteer was immediately assigned to lead me around. Roy was blind but chose not to use a cane. When he sensed he might be getting close to other people, he'd call out, "Beep! Beep!" and hope for the best. He beep-beeped us from my dorm room to the cafeteria to the nurse's office; after that we beep-beeped our way to some classrooms. Each time he insisted on interrupting the teacher. "This is Beth," he'd shout, never apologizing for the disruption. "She's the new student."

Between class visits, Roy told stupid jokes, only partly drowned out by a constant din of questions from my peers in the hallways: "Who's there?" "Where's the doorway?" "Who are you?" "Which way you headed?" All accompanied by the constant tapping of canes. The questions seemed to come from every direction, and they were more unnerving than Roy's jokes. I was relieved when he announced that the guidance counselor's office would be my last stop for the day.

The counselor read my schedule aloud. "There's Braille, home maintenance, daily living skills, typing, career counseling, and . . . let's see . . . oh yes, crafts."

It all sounded OK to me, I said. Mike had joined us, and he gave my hand a squeeze. Getting started in my classes was appealing.

"It's funny, though," she said. "You have a big gap in your schedule every afternoon. Aren't you taking mobility?"

Of course I was taking mobility. Half the reason I was there was to learn how to go places: get on a bus or the El, go up and down curbs, cross busy streets.

I heard fingers fumbling through paper.

"Oh, I see now," she said. "You're not scheduled because your waiver is missing. You need a waiver from your doctor that confirms you're up to the training."

Mike had a better idea of where and how we'd picked up all the documents that constituted my file, so I let him talk. Anyone who has ever been through a paper chase can imagine how it went. Mike says the waiver *must* be there—in fact, he'd taken great pains to get that particular waiver. The guidance counselor says it isn't. Mike asks to look through the file himself; the guidance counselor says he can't. "IVHI Policy," she says. Mike gets angry and says it's our file; the guidance counselor relents. Mike can't find the waiver but insists he gave it to the DORS caseworker in Champaign. The counselor says it must have gotten lost in the mail.

We have to get another waiver before I can start mobility training. In fact, I can't leave the building at all unless a sighted person officially signs me out. "IVHI policy. But don't worry," she coos as she walked us out, "we'll leave your schedule open in the afternoon."

In my head I heard the clang of a cell door slamming behind me. I wasn't at camp; I was in Braille Jail.

"Beth!" Mike hissed in my ear as we stormed down the hallway together. "I *know* we had that waiver. It was the last piece, it was the holdup."

We reached my room. Mike led me through the doorway and continued to grumble. "And then, what do they do? Give you an empty schedule, with a lot of time to pass, which is exactly what we don't want! Which is what you had too much of back at home."

We almost forgot about Roy. Apparently the halls were so noisy that Roy hadn't heard anything Mike said.

"Well," Roy said brightly. I could tell he was smiling. "What do you think?"

I told him I was disappointed that I wasn't scheduled for mobility.

"Oh, no," Roy said. "You can't be disappointed. Well, see you in the morning." I heard the door close.

Mike pressed my head against his shoulder. He let me cry for a while.

"You OK?" he asked finally. I nodded yes as I wiped my face with the back of my hand.

"I don't blame you," Mike said. "You *can't* be disappointed? What kind of attitude is that?"

Mike stayed a while longer, and I promised to call him every night. First thing in the morning he'd go back to the doctor and get a replacement waiver.

It was time for dinner. Mike drew up my insulin, watched me take my shot, and made sure I could get to the cafeteria line by myself. We hugged and kissed goodbye, and I did my best to hold back tears so he wouldn't worry.

As it turned out, Mike had lots more than the tears of separation to worry about. When I called him the next night, I did my best to sound upbeat. But when small talk turned to food and Mike asked what I had eaten for dinner, I had to 'fess up.

"Actually, I didn't eat in the cafeteria tonight," I finally answered.

"You mean you already found someone to get you out of there, take you out for dinner?"

"I wish," I answered. "I didn't eat in the cafeteria because there was no one here to draw up my insulin."

"*What?!*" I could hear him jumping out of his chair. "What about the nurse? Have you eaten yet?"

"Yeah, I ate," I said. "The nurse forgot I was here, though. I guess she was confused—you drew up my insulin last night, so she forgot she had to do it before she went home today."

I explained how I'd tapped my white cane to the nurse's office at four o'clock for my evening insulin, only to find the door locked. There were sighted people around who could have helped, but an administrator insisted that a registered nurse or a licensed physician fill the syringe.

"What about the security guard?" Mike asked. We'd learned the day before that the night security guard was an emergency medical technician.

"He didn't meet the administrator's standards."

"So where did you go?"

"The Cook County Hospital Emergency Room," I answered.

"*Jesus Christ!*" Mike screamed, practically jumping through the phone. He wanted details, but I could barely get a word in as he cursed the administrator, the administrator's mother, and anybody else he could think of.

After he calmed down I explained that I'd been taken to the hospital, put in a wheelchair, parked in a hallway, and told to wait. Two hours passed before someone came to check my blood pressure. Was it always so high, I was asked. Only the day before, the Braille Jail nurse had asked if it was always so *low.* It usually was.

Shortly afterward, a doctor helped me measure my insulin, watched me take my shot, and had me delivered back to Braille Jail.

"They didn't forget about me entirely," I told Mike, trying to reassure him. "They saved a cold tray of food for me."

These little Kafka Meets Cuckoo's Nest episodes pretty much summed up my experience at Braille Jail, although there were a few bright spots. To start, the day after the emergency room debacle, I insisted that the nurse teach me how to measure my insulin injections. It was so simple and low-tech that I had to laugh about all the months I'd relied on Mike simply because no one spent the five minutes to show me the procedure. (Create rows of staples in different lengths, to serve as syringe guides. Put a Braille label on each that indicates the corresponding dosage. Select the proper row of staples; stick the needle into the insulin vial; pull the plunger way back. Shove the row of staples against the syringe. Then push the plunger back down until it hits the staples.)

My cooking instructor was a student teacher who had lost his sight in Vietnam during a practice maneuver. From him I learned how to use special measuring spoons, to measure and pour liquids, even—to Mike's chagrin—how to use a gas range. But how my teacher and I managed day to day without killing each other is still a source of wonder. I'm not good at taking directions, and he corrected me incessantly. It didn't help that, somewhere along the line, I learned he had sideburns like the Las Vegas Elvis and that he wore dated clothes. I realized that he been frozen in fashion time. It was an unnerving thought, and I vowed to avoid that peril myself. Still, I confess that this knowledge helped me through our time together. Whenever he'd nitpick, I'd think, *Oh yeah, well if you're so smart, what's with the muttonchops and bad pants?*

A sighted woman taught the class called "Activities for Daily Living." Among other things, she taught us how to vacuum successfully. "Side to side in parallel lines!" she'd shout over the noise of the Hoover. I imagined her using a megaphone. "Then the same from the other two sides of the room! Like making a checkerboard!" She also taught me how to write checks, address envelopes, and a battery of other skills, but cleaning was what turned her on. "Scrub every surface of the sink, the counters, and the toilet bowl!" she'd exhort, as if she were taping a TV commercial.

My Braille teacher, Pam, was far and away my favorite, an object lesson in dignity and professionalism. She moved into her own place with her guide dog, Sparky, while I was her student. That a single blind person was able to buy her own place was in itself inspirational.

Pam was all business. She'd march into class, tell Sparky to lie down, and ask one of us to read aloud from our Braille books. After critiquing and coaching the first student, she'd ask another, and so on. While one read aloud, the others read silently. Somehow, though we were all at different levels, Pam kept up with every one of us. She took her work very seriously, and she had high standards and expectations. As far as I could tell, she was alone in this regard; as a result, she didn't seem well liked by fellow teachers. I often heard other staff members chatting with Pam, only to make fun of her when she left.

Whether you were a teacher or a student, having high expectations seemed to make you a pariah in the eyes of the Braille Jail staff. Take my crafts class. On our initial tour, Mike and I were told that the school had a kiln. I'd never worked with clay, but pottery sounded appealing. Then, at my first crafts class, I was told that the kiln was broken. "Is there a craft you're already interested in?" the teacher asked. "Shelley over there likes to knit, so she's working on a scarf. And Anita is crocheting."

"I collect rubber stamps," I offered.

"Oh, that's nice," she responded. "Why don't we start you out with belt-making."

I was given a plastic bag of precut leather pieces and a buckle. The teacher showed me how the pieces linked together and let me have at it. After two classes I had produced the belt.

"What's next?" I asked.

She handed me another plastic bag, this time with smaller precut leather pieces and a buckle.

I immediately made my way to the guidance counselor's office.

"Take me out of crafts class," I told her. "It's degrading. There is no reason for me to waste my time making belts when I could be learning how to get around by myself, how to read Braille—"

"Beth," my counselor cut in, "it's a requirement."

She took my hand and put her face close to mine. In a hushed voice she explained, "You know, Beth, we don't provide that class to teach you to make leather belts. We provide it as a time for you to socialize with the other students."

I pulled back. She had bad breath.

"It gives you an atmosphere where you can relax," she continued, "a chance to chat and share your feelings and worries."

I withdrew my hand. "Take me out of that class," I told her. "I can socialize on my own."

I don't know if I was ever officially taken out of crafts class. I simply stopped attending. Not long after that, I was removed from my weekly career counseling class.

The first week a stockbroker came. She was sighted, but both of her parents were blind. With the talking computers that were now available, she thought *maybe* a blind person could be a stockbroker. After explaining a little about what a stockbroker did, she fielded questions. "Do you know any blind people who do this?" I asked. No, she didn't. "Have you ever seen a talking computer read a screen with stocks on it?" No. "Do your parents have a talking computer?" Actually, her parents were at home on Social Security Disability. (Not that any of this was germane to IVHI; in my three months there, the sole talking computer at the school was never in working order.)

The next week an IVHI teacher talked to us about being a rehab teacher. Ditto the following week. After a third consecutive week of in-house speakers, I asked if we were ever going to hear from anyone but IVHI staff.

The instructor took offense. "You don't think being a teacher is a worthwhile career?" he barked.

"Of course I do, but I'd like to hear about some other options."

Our argument ended when he told me that if I didn't like the class the way it was, I shouldn't come back.

And my mobility training? Mike spent a whole day picking up a new blank form, carrying it to the doctor's, and waiting until it was signed. He made a copy, then brought the original on his next weekend visit. On Monday morning I took it straight to my counselor's office.

"I got the form," I announced as I walked in. "Who will be the lucky one to teach me mobility?"

She said she didn't know. "You won't be starting mobility today anyway," she calmly declared. "You have to be seen by our staff doctor. IVHI policy."

"Why didn't you tell me before? I'm killing time every afternoon—I could have had a physical!"

"Our staff doctor has been on vacation since before you arrived."

"And when is he coming back?"

"Not for a couple of weeks," she answered.

Suddenly I imagined that the waiver had always been there, that the whole thing had been a stalling tactic to cover for not having enough instructors. Or who knows? In any case, I didn't start mobility training until just before Thanksgiving. I received less than a month's worth before I made my Christmas escape.

Although I "graduated," the rehab counselors advised against me leaving: I'd had a bad attitude about crafts and socializing; I had learned only rudimentary Braille skills; I was still a bad housekeeper; I had lots more to learn about navigating with a cane. Aside from the socializing, they were all reasonable criticisms. But the way I saw it, I already had friends, I had developed a working knowledge of Braille, I was never a spotless housekeeper, and I could build on my extant mobility skills.

More to the point, I simply hated Braille Jail. It happened to be situated only a few blocks from the same Chicago eye clinic where I had already put in so much time. It meant more driving and weekend only visits for Mike. I was sick of the lengthy absences, and I yearned to be home for Christmas. I decided to bolt and take my chances.

3 | Blind Christmas

At Christmas 1985 I made my blind debut at a major family event. Neither my hospitalizations nor ongoing rehab exempted me from our ritual of drawing a name from a hat and crafting a gift for that person. Pleased with myself, I held out the present I'd built and wrapped myself: a wooden box I'd designed and assembled in my home maintenance class.

"But someone else cut the wood for you, right?" a handy brother-in-law asked.

No, I told him, indignant.

"Really? How did you measure the wood? How did you cut it? You didn't use a saw, I know that!"

I tried to explain how a Braille ruler works. "There are long marks you can feel at every inch," I said, "and smaller ones at the quarter inch. You line it up against the wood and feel the long lines, you count up the inches, then the quarter inches . . ."

But I'd already lost my audience. I heard another conversation starting quietly to my right. On my left, paper crunched. "Who's next?" someone called out. I didn't even get to say that I had, indeed, used a saw.

The next gift was unwrapped and described—for everyone's benefit, not just mine. With six brothers and sisters and all the kids, there are always people far from the action. And, frankly, some of these homemade items are hard to identify with 20-20 eyesight. So things are ritually passed around and admired; when they came my way I held them briefly, running my fingers over the odd contours.

It's a kind of blessing, being part of such a large family. My new blindness wasn't ignored, exactly; it just took a back seat to the usual Christmas chaos. I was happy to let it. Christmas 1985 was typical of how my family deals with major problems: we acknowledge them, then do what's necessary to move on. We don't reflect. We don't analyze. We don't coddle or emote. Not publicly, anyway.

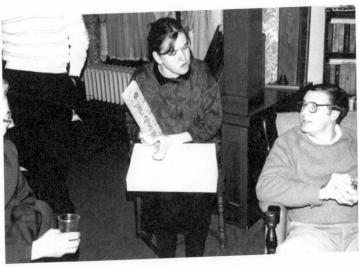

I unwrap and examine, by touch, the mysteries of a homemade Christmas gift.

I've never known another way, so this stoicism seems normal to me. I suppose I could give this a talk-show psychology spin and say we don't express our feelings as well as we should. But it's more of an ethic with us, one that my siblings and I learned from our mother.

Flo has always been unpretentious and uncomplicated to a fault. Once I asked her why she wanted such a large family.

"Well, really," she answered, "I always wanted just two children." Her first-born was my sister Bobbie; the second, my brother Doug. The perfect little family.

"What happened?" I asked.

"Hmmmmm," she said, thinking, then answered with a laugh. "Too many parties, I guess."

———

Flo's farmer grandparents emigrated from Germany in the late 1800s, settling fifteen miles west of Chicago in a town called Elmhurst. The farms had been replaced with postwar housing developments and expressways to the city by the time I was born. The Elmhurst home that Flo and my dad, Eddie Finke, had purchased had been intended for a family of four. By the time I was born, there were no bedrooms left. My crib stood in the hallway until I was two. Finally our family moved to a house with a dry basement, in which Daddy and Uncle Ray built a bedroom for the boys.

Not long after seeing to it that all his children were shoehorned into proper bedrooms, my dad had a heart attack at home. My sister Bev, six years old then, remembers him leaning on the closet door in his bedroom and clutching his chest. I slept through it all. Because I was three at the time, I remember very little about him, and it took years to find out anything else. Every time I asked, someone started crying, so I learned not to ask. Sometimes when we drove by the funeral home I'd call out, "That's where Daddy lives!"

Eventually, Flo went to work. Daddy had switched jobs shortly before his death and had no life insurance. She received Social Security, but it wasn't much. Before I started kindergarten, she took a job at a bakery, where I could go with her. I played and ate fresh bread and doughnuts in the back room while she waited on customers. When I started afternoon kindergarten, one of the other ladies at the bakery walked me to the crossing guard at noon.

My brothers and sisters had already taught me to read, and when my teachers discovered this, they tested me to see if I should skip ahead to first grade. I was tall enough, my test scores were high, and administrators knew my mother would have an easier time of it if I went to school all day. I was promoted at winter break. Flo started taking typing classes in an adult education program and studied for her high school diploma. In 1966, shortly after I turned seven, she took her first full-time job as a clerk at Reliable Electric Company, located twenty minutes away from Elmhurst in an industrial town called Franklin Park. She kept that job for twenty years.

It was during her first summer working that I was diagnosed with diabetes and hospitalized for two weeks. She couldn't miss work, but every morning and evening she'd stop by to see me on her commute. At night she'd leave the hospital early enough to have dinner at home with my sisters. Flo was a single mom, and we younger kids were latchkey children long before those terms were commonplace.

Our oldest brother, Doug, was a talented trombone player. He had been drafted, joined the Marines, and sent us postcards from the different places where he performed with the U.S. Marine Corps Band. Before he left home, he bought the family a piano. I didn't know it then, but later I learned that my father had been a good pianist himself. Now, though it seemed frivolous on her tight budget, Flo made sure we three youngest kids took lessons. Even Beverle, whose childhood dream was to own a drum set, was required to study piano for a year before starting drum lessons at school.

With our other brothers and sisters married or out working, Flo, Marilee, Bev, and I took care of the house, mowed, cleaned out the gutters, did makeshift repairs. The older kids contributed money from their paychecks, Marilee cooked for us, and on Thursday nights (before Flo's payday) we often ate what was left in the refrigerator, usually eggs with toast. But dinner was always ready when Flo arrived home, we never went hungry, and we lived what we considered to be happy, normal lives.

Flo never complained about things being hard or unfair. She *did* complain when we didn't do our chores or if we fought over dishwashing duty or messed up what she'd just finished cleaning. But she never told us we were a burden or that we'd worn her out, though plenty of evenings she just went to her room and lay down. When we went in to ask if anything was wrong, she'd say, "No, I'm just resting my eyes."

Many years later, when I was visiting my son's classroom, another young mother struck up a conversation with me. Eventually we got around to what my childhood had been like.

"Oh, so that's where you get it," she said after I described Flo.

"Get what?"

"Your courage," she answered.

I was flattered but had to chuckle. Flo would have been embarrassed. She didn't believe she was being courageous. She saw her life in simple terms: she did what she had to do. And I realized that I look at my own life that way.

———

My family and I have always handled the big dramas by focusing on the practicalities. For instance, my sister Bobbie simply opened her house to me as I recovered from my second eye surgery. I was happy to have a place to visit with people where I didn't feel pressed to entertain them. It was a special treat that my sister Marilee happened to be in town with her two children during my recovery; Marilee's husband was in the military, and they would move to Germany that fall.

Marilee was a gawky twelve-year-old with braces and glasses back in 1966 when Flo started working full-time. It was Marilee who cooked our dinners and kept the house clean. She never participated in after-school activities and was always there when Bev and I got home from school. My older siblings say Marilee was born this way—never any trouble, always someone you could rely on.

I was a gawky twelve-year-old myself, likewise with braces and glasses, when Marilee hugged me goodbye and left for college in 1971. By then her contact lenses revealed beautiful dark brown eyes. Her hair had that same rich brown color, and her smile showcased straight, white teeth. She majored in elementary education, and I was sure she was the prettiest student teacher at her school. Her metamorphosis from duckling to swan gave me hope.

Marilee's company alone would have been enough to improve my days in the lounge chair, but, like my other sisters, she waited on me, too—reading books and articles aloud, feeding me my meals so I wouldn't have to lift my head. She taught her preschool son Robbie to bring me a can of soda with an elbow straw, and her daughter Jennifer enjoyed guiding me to the bathroom, giggling every time I asked her to place my hand on the toilet paper.

Another sister, Cheryl, visited often, usually bringing Flo. Flo and Cheryl are more like sisters than mother and daughter, both in manner and in looks. While the rest of us are tall and straight like our dad, Flo and Cheryl are short and round. Both still lived in Elmhurst, minutes from Bobbie's home in Downers Grove. Cheryl readily admits she wanted her three children to grow up as she had, and she was tickled whenever someone told her she was "just like her mother." It was Cheryl who had realized how terribly much I must miss being home after that last month in the hospital. She's the one who'd volunteered to drive me down to Champaign and haul me back to a doctor's appointment in Chicago a few days later, though it meant that her husband, a fireman, had to take time off from work to watch their kids.

Mike has always been the first to point out that while I was losing my sight, and later adapting to blindness, the nuts-and-bolts help my family offered was invaluable. All the same, he sometimes views my family—and to some extent me—with ambivalence, even astonishment. He was as happy as I was when no one made a fuss about my blindness that first Christmas. "It was nice to forget about all of it," he told me later, "to not have it be the most important thing." Yet he could also say, "But Beth, doesn't it seem like someone would take you aside and ask, 'How you doing?' or 'What's it like?' or *something*?"

His own family was much more circumscribed—mother, father, one sister, no extended family close by. So he's always been a little intimidated by the sheer bulk of my family. As he's fond of saying, "It isn't a family, it's a freaking nation." Size wasn't the only difference. His mother was the oldest of three daughters of Italian immi-

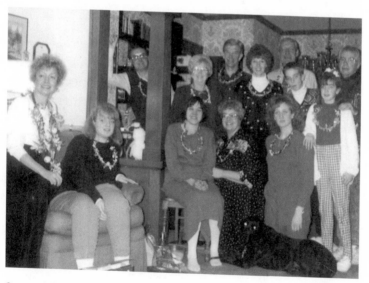

Some of the Finkes, attired in homemade neckwear, at a holiday gathering, 1991.

grants, vastly more colorful and expressive than any of the Finkes. She loved politics, current events, sports—she had an intense combative streak. Mike's father was a different story. Also born to immigrants (Serbian), Mike's dad was one of seven children. He and his three brothers served in World War II but rarely spoke about the war. Mike's dad had a kind, easy-going demeanor that would have allowed him to blend contentedly into my family's big communal gatherings. Mike and I often laugh about the similarities between his dad and my mom. Both seemed to subscribe to a creed of "Be nice, have fun, and above all, avoid controversy." So his parents were polar opposites, and his challenge has been to balance traits inherited from them both. The father part embraces my family; the mother part makes him want to leap up and run screaming.

———

Anyway, that's how it was at my first blind Christmas. After all the gift-giving, I went through the buffet line on Mike's arm. "There's seven-layer salad, potato salad, turkey, ham, deviled eggs, cookies, stuffing, some green globby-looking stuff, and Jell-O," he blurted without a breath. "What'll it be?" It was always the same: Flo made German potato salad, Cheryl always brought seven-layer salad, Bobbie the spinach and cheese casserole. I knew *exactly* what was on the table.

"OK, lots of seven-layer salad," I told him, "and give me some of the green globby stuff." Mike filled both our plates and balanced them beautifully while steering me to a folding chair. I managed to eat and drink without spilling.

"Can I take this for you?" Mike asked when he saw I was done.

"I dunno," I answered, "there any seven-layer salad left?"

"You want *more*?" Mike asked. If it weren't so hard to get exercise without being able to see, blind people would all be very, very skinny. When you have to make an announcement every time you want a second helping, you tend to eat less.

"Well, yeah," I admitted. He harrumphed, headed off with my plate, came right back saying the seven-layer was history. "You want anything else?"

"Skip it," I said, not wanting him to bother. He left again. When I heard Flo call out, "Save the plastic! Save the plastic!" I realized he must have headed to the garbage can with my plate. Big mistake. Flo has an obsession about reusing things.

Mike sat next to me again and I teased him, "That wasn't you trying to throw out the plastic forks, was it?"

"Jesus Christ!" he said, "What's with that?"

"Well, *honey*," I said, doing my best Junior Leaguer imitation while rubbing his thigh under the vinyl-covered table, "Flo likes to recycle."

"So do I, but why doesn't she just use regular silverware? The whole point of plastic is that it's *disposable*."

"Well, yeah, but Flo isn't most people."

"Don't they melt in the dishwasher?"

"Oh, Mike, come on! Flo doesn't own a dishwasher. She washes everything by hand."

There was also the ritual of arranging the cars in the driveway. Earlier Flo had reminded everyone (as always) that they ticket you for parking in the street.

"She thinks you get an FBI record for a parking ticket?" Mike asked in an exasperated whisper. "One day I'm going to leave my car in the street *all night*, just to make everyone crazy." I laughed, knowing that my glee would only egg him on.

"And what's with the clocks in this house? They're all ten minutes fast."

"That's so we're never late," I explained.

"Beth, you're *always* late. Besides, you *know* that the clocks are fast."

"Works for us," I said.

After dinner I spent the rest of my first blind Christmas evening as I always had: camped at the dining room table drinking coffee, telling stories, laughing with my sisters. Mike sat right there with us, listening, making fun of us, gathering ammunition to make me laugh the next day. True to family form, no one asked about white canes or Braille.

A decade would pass before I would learn that each family member had grieved privately when they heard I wouldn't see again.

Bev, living in Texas at the time, lay on a raft in her backyard pool and looked up at the blue sky. "Beth can't see this," she said to herself, then started to cry.

For some reason it hit Cheryl as she gardened. "I started thinking of you and burst into tears," she told me. Cheryl is not particularly religious, but she left her tomatoes right then and walked to a nearby church to pray with the pastor. "I was all full of mud and dirt," she said. "He didn't even know who I was. He must have thought I was nuts."

My brother Doug was afraid to talk to me that Christmas, he admitted later. "I thought I'd offend or upset you. I didn't want to say the wrong thing." Truth is, in the din of family Christmas cheer that day, I never noticed his silence.

With my sister Bobbie things were a little different. She and her husband, Harry, had been closer to my medical saga than the others. After we'd gotten the bad news from my eye surgeon, Mike called her from the baseball game to say we wouldn't be returning to her house that evening, so she'd been the first to learn I was blind. But then Bobbie didn't need the full explanation; she understood my condition, the medical details, and what had been at stake all along.

I'm twenty years younger than Bobbie. For a long time she seemed as much like an aunt as she did a sister. But when she was diagnosed with Type 1 diabetes at the age of twenty-eight, a bond began to develop between us. We sort of became our own support group of two.

I didn't think much about it at the time, but it couldn't have been

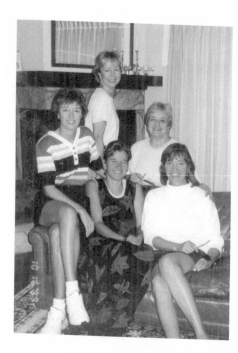

The Finke sisters (clock-
wise from top): Bobbie,
Cheryl, Marilee, Beth,
and Beverle, 1999.

easy for her to stay so close to me as I was losing my sight. The risk
of diabetic complications grows the longer one has had the disease.
So when she visited me at the hospital, when I lay (face-down, of
course) on that chaise on her backyard deck, when she got the news
from Mike, she must have wondered about her own fate. If she did,
she never let on.

And as for Flo, I've never asked about how she took the news,
and she's never offered.

That Christmas night, the only thing out of the ordinary was the
attention I got when my coffee ran out or I needed another pack of
Sweet 'n' Low. As the youngest, I was used to getting some extra attention, but nothing like this. As with my diabetes diagnosis when I
was a kid, this new situation evoked no pity, just the added dollop
of care and concern. I enjoyed it.

We stayed over at my mom's that night, as did a couple of my sisters and their families, so there was plenty of help if I needed it. I'd grown up in that house, though; I knew it so well that I didn't even need my cane. Mike and I slept soundly, and our breakfast announcement that we'd be returning to Champaign that day was met with a chorus of protests.

"Aren't you coming downtown with us to eat by the tree at Marshall Field's?" Flo asked. "We do that every year. You have to come."

"We didn't go sledding yet, Aunt Beth!" one of the nieces whined. "You have to stay until we go sledding."

I took their protests as a good sign. It never occurred to them that I might not get much out of a trip to Marshall Field's or that sledding might be problematic. I was the same good old Aunt Beth to them.

"Thanks," I said to Flo, "but I think I've spent enough time in Chicago this year; I'll skip Marshall Field's."

"But what about sledding?" my niece asked. I could feel her standing next to my knees. I lifted her onto my lap. "Awww, Stacey," I said, "I'd love to go. But you can go without me."

"But it's more fun if you go."

My youngest nieces and nephews have been consistently unbothered, even entertained, by my condition. A four-year-old nephew once showed me a picture. "See me?" he asked, rubbing my hand back and forth over the photo. I eventually learned to play a game in which they'd bring me household objects and ask me to identify them. They were rarely able to stump me, and I learned that small children are an easy audience. All seemed to take pride in serving as my sighted guides, though Mike disapproves of this practice, especially after that time he witnessed a seven-year-old niece leading me head-on into a light pole. The teenagers in the family have always been forthright about the way blindness changed my actions and looks. I've appreciated their candor—brutal as it's been at times—because I haven't always been able to count on the same honesty from adults. One of my fears after losing my sight was that I'd get frozen in a fashion time warp, like my cooking teacher at Braille Jail. So while comments like, "Aunt Beth, you look like a dork!" or "How come you're wearing that dumb scarf?" might have lacked tact, I welcomed them.

It was from Cheryl's youngest daughter, Caren, that I first learned one of my eyes had reached the point of outright gruesomeness. Some time had passed since my surgeries, and I was visiting Flo for a few days. Caren wasn't old enough to have a job, so she dropped over often to keep me company. She was a typically awkward adolescent, but still completely comfortable hanging out with me, white cane and all. The two of us traipsed all over Elmhurst. If people stared at us, she didn't seem to notice or care. But on one of our strolls, as we blabbed about TV shows and her school friends, she blurted out of nowhere, "Aunt Beth, your eye is really ugly."

My hand flew to my face. I had forgotten my sunglasses. Of course I no longer needed to protect my sight, but I still wore them to conceal my right eye. Surgical trauma had caused it to shrink, and I could barely hold it open. Evidently whatever still showed was quite disturbing. I asked Caren for details.

"Well, it's just weird-looking." she said, "red and bloody and gross."

That was all I needed. When we got back to Flo's, I immediately phoned Mike and confronted him.

"Does my eye look gross?" I demanded. "And if it does, why didn't you tell me?"

I'd caught him a little off balance. He hesitated, then admitted that my eye did look "beat up," but that he really didn't notice it anymore. "Besides," he said, "it's the least of our worries."

It quickly became the first of mine. Not long after that I contacted an ocularist, who eventually fitted me with a prosthesis so genuine-looking that even Caren couldn't tell it wasn't real.

I suppose those of us who have what we consider happy family lives take them for granted. But isn't that as it should be? I know that as I lost my sight, as I adapted to being blind, and later when our son was born, I really needed to be able to take *something* for granted. I am so fortunate that I could.

4 | Gus

Since our wedding, what with eye surgeries and Braille Jail, Mike and I had slept apart more than we'd slept together. We shared responsibility for birth control. One time he'd be in charge; the next time I would. More often than not, we both used something. Diabetics are better off avoiding the pill, so when it was my turn, I used a diaphragm. Mike, of course, used a condom. That evening was Mike's turn. As a welcome-home present, he'd bought an extra-special type, advertised as "so much like your own skin, you can hardly tell you have it on."

The advertisement didn't lie. We could hardly tell it was on. Or off.

We both had a strong sense we were in trouble. This time, naturally, we hadn't doubled up on protection. I didn't know how early you could go to the doctor to see if you were pregnant, and home pregnancy tests were still in the future. Besides, the notion of being pregnant was just too much to contemplate. So I spent my days applying my newly learned skills, re-connecting with friends, and just being home with Mike.

During my hospitalizations Mike had managed to keep working on various contract writing projects, but when we learned I wouldn't see again, he tied up loose ends and stopped taking on new work. When I left for Braille Jail, he began sniffing out new projects again, but the previous contract jobs had dried up. By the end of the holidays he had still found nothing.

Which was fine by me. It was so good being together in our own place again. Money was tight, but we weren't desperate. We'd managed to save a little while we were both working, and I continued to receive half my regular salary on temporary disability from the university. Also, shortly after we were married, we'd moved into a campus apartment that was dirt cheap. Years earlier I'd put my name on a waiting list while still a student. I'd actually forgotten about it when the call came. We'd miss our Urbana rental house, but what we'd save could eventually go toward buying our own place. We took a one-bedroom unit for $135 a month, including utilities. That decision turned out to be a lifesaver.

Then again, maybe you get what you pay for. Only a couple of weeks after my escape from Braille Jail, we were awakened early by three sharp knocks: "There's a fire in the basement!" shouted the apartment manager. "You have to *get out!*"

We could already smell smoke. Years earlier I had grabbed my photo albums during a fire alarm in my college dorm. This time I felt around for my clothes and reached across our dresser for a jar of change.

I called out for Mike.

"I'm right here," he shouted. "I have your coat. Grab my arm."

I could hear fire trucks coming as we rushed outside and crossed the street. We met most of our neighbors for the first time as we stood watching (or smelling, in my case) the burning building. The old boiler had malfunctioned, setting the basement on fire. Eventually we were told we couldn't go back inside until at least that afternoon.

I felt pretty proud of myself for grabbing that jar of change. I held it up and shook it in front of Mike.

"Hey, you wanna go out for breakfast?" Over bacon and eggs we decided to call our friends Anne and Billy to alert them that we needed a place to stay warm for the day.

I had been friends with Anne since college. She and Billy had met in 1982, when she and I were killing time at a bar, waiting for a new crop of British students to arrive from O'Hare. (It was part of my job to greet incoming exchange students and to deliver them to their new American dorm rooms.) Always game for new experiences, Anne agreed to stay up late with me and wait for them. Billy was at the bar that night, and he took a quick interest in Anne.

The two of them had lived together before getting married, and their wedding had been small and simple. The party weeks later was a different story. Anne had met her match in Billy; they had hundreds of friends, many coming from far away to join the celebration.

Mike and I were still at Anne and Billy's place when they returned from work that night. And every night for three weeks. Besides the boiler, which was destroyed, there had been only smoke damage and smashed doors. (The firemen had battered them as they checked each apartment.) But city inspectors found code violations, so things dragged out. We were grateful for a safe haven, and Anne was happy for the company on the many nights when Billy worked late. We all managed to make the best of it, with what could have been a disaster turning into a long slumber party.

——— ———

We returned home again and instantly realized it had been more than a month since our contraceptive fiasco. My period was overdue. Camping out with our friends had made it easy to ignore the subject; now we could think of nothing else. I called my doctor and Mike took me in the same day for a blood test. The nurse instructed us to call the next afternoon for results.

Luckily my appointment with Janet Floyd at the Rehab Center was also the next day, giving me something to do besides fret. When I'd first gone to her, I was still thinking my eyesight would return. Now I was ready to listen. Janet explained how blind people were routinely accepted into University of Illinois graduate programs; supported by the Rehab Center, they completed master's and other professional degrees. She reeled off the names of past students: one a computer programmer, another a counselor, another a lawyer.

When she asked if I had any interest in graduate study, I said I might like to be a counselor. She liked that idea. In fact, she was part of a group designing a new master's program in something called Rehabilitation Counseling. If it was approved, I could be in the very first class.

"Geez, Beth," Mike laughed when he picked me up, "what's put the bounce in your step?" He helped me into the car. I couldn't stop talking. The idea of starting something new, and succeeding, had me a little giddy. "So when would you start? Next fall?"

I said yes. "There's no reason a blind woman couldn't be a counselor, right? In fact, it might be an advantage—I'd have to judge clients by what they say instead of how they look."

"I suppose so," Mike said, then changed the subject. The apartment was freezing, the new boiler still not up to speed. He suggested stopping by campus for a cup of coffee to warm up before going home.

As we drove to the Union, I heard a radio DJ announce the time. "Four-thirty already? God, I forgot!" I burst out. "I still have to call the lab. It closes at five."

"We'll call from the Union," Mike offered.

My thoughts instantly switched from graduate school to babies, and that ignited a mixed bag of emotions. I couldn't imagine caring for a baby now. In fact, I'd never considered what it would be like to have a baby under any circumstances. Pregnancy, I knew, could cause or accelerate diabetic complications. But the complication I had feared most was blindness, so what did I have to lose? Like graduate school, a baby could be something positive, something offering hope. Having a baby lets you call people with *good* news. If I were pregnant, maybe I could make some sense out of losing my sight. Maybe we'd produce a Nobel Prize winner, someone who'd find the cure for cancer. Or diabetes.

But what about graduate school? Or returning to work? I was still having trouble walking around the block without falling off curbs. I certainly wasn't ready to tackle graduate school plus work plus motherhood.

I finally decided that no matter what the test showed, I would view it as good news. If it turned out I wasn't pregnant, we'd consider it a lucky escape and I'd start getting paperwork together for graduate school. If I was pregnant, Mike and I would have a happy project to work on, raising our Nobel Prize winner.

— —

My voice shook as I asked for absolute clarification. "Positive means I am pregnant, right?"

What a strange feeling. I was anxious and scared but couldn't stop grinning.

When the voice on the phone confirmed, I covered the mouthpiece, turned toward Mike and whispered, "I'm pregnant." This was one of those moments that I have experienced hundreds, maybe thousands of times since: I needed to see Mike's face, but I couldn't.

No time to dwell on that, though—I had to choose an obstetrician. I repeated names and phone numbers aloud so Mike could write them down. When I hung up at last, I immediately called for an appointment with my physician, an endocrinologist who specialized in diabetes. I'd read enough books, been to enough seminars, to know it was extremely important, for me and the baby, that the doctor check me immediately. The receptionist told me he couldn't see me for a week. I reminded her I was a pregnant diabetic. Didn't matter, she said, the doctor had no openings until next week. We called another clinic and got an appointment for the next day. I never saw my old doctor again.

"You don't think I'm nuts?" I asked my new specialist. "A blind diabetic having a kid?"

"If you are healthy right now, willing to check your blood sugar levels four, five, and maybe six times a day, plus come here weekly for tests throughout the pregnancy, and—most important—you decide you want to have this baby," he said, taking a deep breath, "there is absolutely no reason why you can't."

"And if we decide we don't want to go through with the pregnancy?" Mike asked.

"I know a very good doctor in town who performs abortions. If you need it, I'll give you her name and number. I can even call her for you if you'd like."

We nodded.

"But, since there is a chance you'll continue the pregnancy, we have to start multiple daily blood tests. And you have to go from here directly to the lab so we can assess your current health."

Among other things, he wanted to check my kidney function. Like the eyes, kidneys are vulnerable in diabetics. Mine had always tested fine, but if there was even the hint of an existing problem, pregnancy would be extremely dicey—carrying a baby puts added stress on any woman's kidneys. A glycosylated hemoglobin test was the other critical component to making this decision. It would indicate how my blood sugars had been over the past three months. Sugar levels at the time of conception and early in the pregnancy are critical: the higher they are, the greater the chance of certain birth defects and other complications.

On the way downstairs to the lab, Mike and I decided we'd go through with the tests and take it from there. "If the results are bad," Mike said, "you have to get an abortion. I don't want things getting any worse for you, Beth."

"But if they're good?"

"Then we'll have to decide."

Part of me wanted the test to save us from making that decision.

In the meantime, I was put on three injections a day, up from two. Weekly appointments with a nutritionist and a health educator were scheduled. If we chose to go ahead, the blood tests and weekly appointments would continue throughout the pregnancy, on top of whatever the obstetrician might require.

When I told Mike before we got married that I shouldn't have children, he accepted the news. Fatherhood wasn't on top of his list of priorities, he said, and if we later changed our minds, we could try to adopt. But back then it was all hypothetical. The reality of pregnancy turned everything inside out, and we were both caught off guard by the exciting prospect of parenthood.

By any rational measure, the idea was nuts. There was my health; the increased odds of a birth defect or other problems for the baby; Mike's current unemployment; my blindness. We knew all that. But we hadn't had any good surprises for a long time. Things hadn't worked out as we had intended, to put it mildly. We hashed it over a million ways, trading roles as we debated. The hand-wringing went on for days.

"Ah, let's do it!" Mike finally exclaimed, his voice a contradictory mix of exasperation and excitement. He added one caveat: "As long as you're healthy."

I still wasn't sure. Days earlier I'd been completely sold on going back to work and starting graduate school. Those prospects still appealed to me. Also, I was strangely concerned about what I'd look like. I already felt like a spectacle every time I stepped outside with my white cane, and I could only imagine the glares I'd get when I was pregnant. ("Look at her! She can't even find a mailbox, and she has the audacity to think she can be a mother?") I wondered how I could tap the cane correctly with a big belly in front of me, and I wasn't at all sure I wanted to learn. But I knew that somehow I'd be able to care for a baby. I trusted myself to figure out the specifics when I had to.

"We'd be great parents." Mike said, interrupting my thoughts, "and I think our kid would be very interesting."

Mike's enthusiasm was contagious. Before I knew it, I found that big smile on my face again, the same one I had right after hanging up the pay phone in the Union.

"But the minute we get any bad test results on you or the baby—" Mike said. It became his mantra.

As it happened, that week marked the thirteenth anniversary of the Supreme Court's *Roe v. Wade* decision. Protesters were out in force at the local abortion clinic. It made me furious—and scared— to think I might have to pass through that swarm of zealots in order to save my own health. "I'll be with you," Mike assured me. "I'll

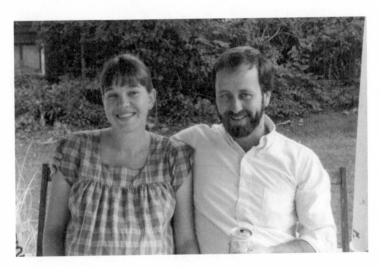

Mike and I sit on our porch swing during my pregnancy, 1986.

kill 'em if they get near you. What the hell do they know about *life*? What the hell do they know about *us*?" Well, Mike gets carried away—he'd never kill anybody, not even someone trying to block my entry to a clinic.

But there would be no such confrontation. My test results were all fine. We chose to proceed with the pregnancy.

———   ———

I put the graduate school applications aside and turned my full attention to practicing the daily living skills I'd learned at Braille Jail. I wanted to be confident by the time the baby arrived. If it arrived. Throughout my pregnancy, I was prepared for the worst; I practically expected it. But just in case things went right, I wanted to be ready.

As for working, that decision turned out to have been made for me. When I was investigating graduate school options, I inquired about a tuition waiver—free tuition was a perk for university employees. I learned I was no longer eligible for the waiver because I was no longer an employee. My contract had been terminated, and I'd been bumped to permanent disability. All without so much as a word from my old boss.

I was angry. More than that, I was hurt. Even though it would be four years before the Americans with Disabilities Act (ADA) was passed, I still could have sued. A lawyer later told us that, under certain labor laws, a person must be given formal notice—usually a letter in the mail—when a contract is terminated. Mike's "Beth file" is jammed with medical bills, Department of Rehabilitation forms, and health insurance booklets. That file even contains the letter stating that I am eligible for Social Security Disability benefits, but no letter about my contract being terminated.

Letter or no letter, I had enough on my plate. I let it be.

Had I lost my job after 1990, when the ADA was passed, I still might not have sued. The burden of proof in a discrimination case is placed on the blind person, and court cases are lengthy and expensive. Still, after 1990 I doubt that I would have been fired in the first place. I can only speculate, but since the Americans with Disabilities Act has spotlighted both the plight and the rights of disabled workers, the mere threat of an ADA lawsuit, with its ensuing bad publicity, might have been enough to keep me employed.

Mike finally received a job offer, but it would require working on the other side of town, so he wouldn't have enough time to come home and perform my noon blood test. Again Anne came to our rescue, volunteering to swing by during her lunch break; this despite being deathly afraid of needles. I eventually resolved to make things a little easier by getting to her office by myself. I learned a route I could navigate safely with my white cane, and this little triumph boosted my confidence. Then in August we moved again—our cheap little apartment wouldn't do for a family of three, and besides, management didn't allow children. Coincidentally, our old rental house in Urbana came vacant. We moved back, and Anne resumed her original routine, traveling to our new place every day for lunchtime blood tests.

Controlling diabetes under normal circumstances is tricky, but during my first trimester, my body became a sort of biochemical cauldron. Hormonal changes produced inexplicably erratic blood sugar levels that dictated frequent alterations in my diet plan and in my thrice-daily doses of insulin. Low blood sugars came faster and harder; we kept candy bars in each room of the house and never left home without sugary treats in our pockets.

Our lives were consumed by my quest for good blood sugars. Every morning I'd prick my finger before lifting my head from the pillow; Mike would bring the glucometer to the bedside for a fasting test. We'd calculate the results to determine my morning dose of insulin, eat breakfast together, and Mike would test my blood again before leaving for work.

While we still lived in the apartment, my mornings were spent fiddling around. We had stored my upright piano at a friend's place (it never made the move to our second-floor apartment) but I had that violin from Mike, and I continued with lessons. Before removing the instrument from its case, I'd listen for footsteps on the stairs in an attempt to verify that most of our neighbors had left the building. Though I practiced each day, I never seemed to improve much.

Anne arrived before noon for my pre-lunch test. (Her friend Nancy served as backup if Anne couldn't make it.) The fiddle was safely stashed away long before she arrived; I didn't want anyone catching me in the midst of scratching and squeaking. Anne would smear the blood on a stick, announce the reading, and record it in our logbook. Before leaving, she'd check my syringe to make sure I'd drawn out the correct amount. Two afternoons each week—and later on in the pregnancy, three afternoons—were spent at the clinic for lab tests or appointments with diabetes educators, nutritionists, obstetricians, endocrinologists. Mike wasn't allowed time off from work, so friends were recruited to drive me. Mike made dinner when he got home, calculating protein, fat and carbohydrate levels with the same precision we used to determine insulin doses. He tested my blood before we ate and again afterward. Once the dishes were done, he phoned the endocrinologist at home to give the day's blood sugar readings. The doctor used these statistics to determine changes in insulin and diet for the next day. We'd go to bed then, but not before doing—you guessed it—one last blood test.

With all its chaos, pregnancy granted me a share of unexpected benefits. For one thing, I felt great. No morning sickness, and with such tight blood-sugar control I began to sense what it must be like to have a working pancreas. For another, I learned a lot more about the nutritional value of what I ate—I became adept at making fine judgments about how quickly certain foods raised my blood sugar level and how much counteracting insulin to take. Such lessons serve me to this day. But if another life hadn't been involved, if the program hadn't been limited to nine months, I couldn't have lived as I did. There was no spontaneity—I couldn't exercise harder than I'd planned, eat more or less than prescribed, or vary my daily routine without my doctor's blessing. All in all, my pregnancy went extraordinarily well.

Our little fetus was doing fine, too. Certain birth defects are more common among babies born to diabetic mothers, and my obstetrician ordered tests for those. We went to a hospital in Chicago to see if the baby's heart was OK. It was. We had a test to make sure the baby didn't have spina bifida or any other neural tube defect. It didn't. We knew early on that our baby would be born by Caesarean section. Diabetic babies are larger than normal, and once they develop to the point where they can survive outside the womb, it's best to deliver them.

Judging from my girth, our baby seemed more likely to win a prizefight than a Nobel Prize. I wasn't due until late September, but in August my obstetrician brought up the possibility of amniocentesis.

Dr. Fay was in her late twenties, like us. "She looks like she's about nineteen!" Mike would laugh. She was enthusiastic and clearly cared about her patients, lavishing time on each. Knowing I'd receive that same sort of thoughtful concern when it came my turn, I didn't mind waiting.

Amniocentesis involved some danger because amniotic fluid is removed with a needle. We finally opted against it for several reasons. The fetus was already big and the amount of amniotic fluid proportionally small; my blood-sugar control was as good as it had ever been; earlier tests had already ruled out diabetes-related birth defects.

Partly because we didn't have the amnio, visits to the clinic for fetal monitoring became more frequent as the due date approached. On September 3, 1986, Dr. Fay noticed a change in the fetus and decided delivery should occur right away. I asked if I could go home for my stuff.

She told me she'd schedule my Caesarean for one o'clock that afternoon, "So come back by noon and check in."

How odd it seemed, making an appointment to have a baby. I waited until I was home to call Mike. I heard panic in his voice.

"I thought I was ready for this," he said, excitement suddenly overtaking the panic. "It's really going to happen!"

During the short drive to the hospital we started facing the fact that we hadn't settled on a name. Mike's mom, Esther, had teased that we should combine her name with my mom's, Florence, to make Florescence. I honestly liked it, at least for a middle name if it was a girl. Mike disagreed.

"What if it's a boy?" I asked in the car. Mike had a favorite uncle named George, so that was a possibility. There were Mike's favorite baseball players. But Roberto Knezovich or Carlton Knezovich? Nah.

Then there was Gus, my father's father's name. He was the sweet quiet grandpa everyone in the family loved. He died in 1963, a year after my dad. I'd always suggested the name Gus for new babies in my family. It was a joke, really—I knew it was never in the running. But on the ride to the hospital it ceased to be a joking matter. We decided that if the baby was a boy, we'd name him Gus.

———   ———

We checked in and I was scrubbed and prepped for surgery. It felt so different from my eye surgeries: this time I was hopeful, not consumed by dread, only worried about the spinal block I'd be given. I wouldn't feel the bottom half of my body during the surgery. What if something went wrong? I couldn't handle being blind and stuck in a wheelchair for the rest of my life. But there was no alternative, and this anxiety passed.

My body was bisected by a little curtain. Mike sat by my shoulders, only my upper torso visible to him. He rested his camera in his lap and rubbed my forehead. I heard a sound like a drill and began to smell something. "What's burning?" I asked. He didn't answer right away; the noises, the nauseating smells from behind the curtain were getting to him. It didn't help to learn that they were coming from an instrument that was cauterizing my tissue. As he grew lightheaded, he instinctively stood and peeked over the curtain. Somehow, seeing it was a relief.

"It's your skin," he said, marveling at what he was watching. "They're cutting you open."

The mechanical noises stopped and I heard what sounded for all the world like a cork being slowly, carefully withdrawn from a champagne bottle. My baby was being lifted out of my uterus. Then a pinched squeak that sounded vaguely like a baby's cry, and someone announced, "It's a boy!"

The room fell frighteningly silent for a moment. Then all hell seemed to break loose, loud fast talk and the sound of footsteps rushing back and forth.

"What's happening?" I asked Mike. Either he was crying or just couldn't speak. "I don't know," he finally answered. "They have him on a machine or something, and there's a bunch of doctors and nurses around him."

Dr. Fay interrupted with a question. "In light of what's going on, do you still want to go ahead with the tubal ligation?" Mike and I had agreed that this pregnancy would be my last.

I didn't *know* what was going on, but whatever it was, I was all the more sure I wanted my tubes tied.

Mike must have concurred. We spontaneously chorused "Yes!"

While Dr. Fay finished my surgery, other doctors and nurses worked on Gus. For some reason, all I could think of was Mike's camera sitting there, unused.

———   ———

Do they have funerals for newborn babies? I wondered as I lay in the recovery room. *Do they have tiny caskets, or do they just dispose of their bodies like so much medical waste?*

I heard a voice. It was Russ, our friend from those U of I basketball games. Earlier that morning Russ had considered himself a lucky guy: it had been his turn to take me to the fetal monitoring session on the very day the baby would be born. He decided to stay on for the big event. Now he was present for the crisis.

"Are you all right?" he asked, grabbing my hand with both of his. I shook my head no. I had the shivers. He left and soon a nurse brought in another blanket. I rocked myself back and forth.

Mike came in and we were introduced to Dr. Ionnides, Gus's neonatal specialist, who told us Gus might have contracted an infection in the womb. There were definitely problems with Gus's heart, he said, and they'd ordered a helicopter to take him to Peoria, where a hospital had a cardiac unit for newborns.

Still woozy, I thought, *Maybe this is somebody I can ask about funerals.* I didn't, but the image of that tiny casket floated in my mind. *Do you have a private funeral? Does a preacher have to be there? Would people understand our grief, or would they think our loss was a blessing?*

I drifted in and out. I heard familiar voices but couldn't tell if they were real. And there were definite hospital noises: beeps, squeaky wheels, the shuffle of soft-soled shoes. Suddenly my funeral obsession was displaced by a powerful sensation of—I don't know what to call it. Peace? *Maybe I'm dying,* I thought. But I knew I wasn't. I felt somehow that a lot of people were thinking of us, all at the same time. I don't know what the trendy word for it is now, but back then it was "vibes," and they were good and strong.

This interlude was interrupted by Dr. Ionnides's return to my bedside. "We're not sure how it happened," he explained, "but the baby's condition has reversed itself." The immediate crisis was over and the helicopter had been canceled. "He's still in trouble, though," he warned us. His voice was flat and serious, with a Greek accent. "I have to tell you his chances are less than fifty-fifty."

Gus had been admitted into the hospital's neonatal intensive care unit. "If he doesn't make it, we tried," I told Mike after Dr. Ionnides had left the room. I was still dopey from the painkiller, but I knew what I was saying. "We did a wonderful job, we gave him a great chance, and we'll go on." We talked about our future, with or without Gus. I truly believe we were prepared to lose him.

I was wheeled to a room, but not one of those doubles in the maternity ward. It was a single in the gynecological surgery wing, far away from the happy mothers with healthy infants. (Years later I learned that this reassignment was common practice—as was the marking of my name in red on the patient list behind the nurse's desk, reminding staff not to gush good wishes when entering my room.)

Anne and Nancy visited, having left their signature kazoos and balloons at home. I heard their footsteps as they entered, but neither spoke. For months they'd been reading aloud to me from books about prenatal care, about naming the baby, about bathing and nursing and what to expect as the child grows. There was no chapter about sick babies, none titled "When Things Go Horribly Wrong."

Anne finally managed to break the awkward silence. Trying her best to sound upbeat, she forced out a "Congratulations!"

Mike's sister Kris visited with her son Aaron, but they weren't allowed inside the intensive care nursery. "Only immediate family members," the head nurse scolded. Anne and Nancy went down and tried to peek through the window. Back in my room, Nancy offered the obligatory "He's cute." Her words were as absurd as Anne's congratulations. Even if she'd been able to get anywhere near Gus, he was so covered with high-tech gear it would have been impossible to tell what his skin color was, much less judge what his face looked like.

For two days I refused to be wheeled down to the neonatal intensive care nursery. If I spent time with Gus, I knew I'd become attached. Then I'd have to grieve even more when they told me he was dead.

Mike visited Gus as often as allowed. He usually asked me to go along but never pressured me. I used the excuse that I wouldn't be able to touch Gus anyway, what with the wires and tubes. "You can touch one leg," Mike answered, trying to encourage me. Gus's left leg was apparently the only part of him not bandaged or connected to one device or another.

A special irony was his shaved head. Before he'd been born, I hadn't cared whether he was a boy or a girl. Beyond the obvious wish for good health, all I hoped for was a baby with a full head of hair I could touch. I got what I wanted. Gus had been born with hair, brown and curly, I learned, but it had been buzzed off so electrodes could be attached to his scalp.

Aside from Mike, the only people who touched Gus in his first days of life were medical experts. I was content to stay railed in bed, partly due to the chemicals available there. Doctors had prescribed intravenous Demerol, complete with a little clicker that let me dose myself. Every ten minutes I could have more; all I had to do was press. And press I did. Moments later a warm glow would start at my forehead and inch down my whole body. I'd forget about the baby, my pain, and even my blindness. In fact, during those first few minutes after a new dose, I could see again—I saw myself from above, looking down, a body in a bed. Then, too soon, I'd crash back into myself and start asking what time it was, counting the minutes until I could hit the clicker.

Mike was stuck with the real world. He had to go back to work the day after my delivery. Each afternoon when his shift was done he came immediately to the hospital, splitting his time between my room and the intensive care nursery, doting first on me, then on Gus.

On the third day of my standoff I was finally shamed into taking the trip to meet my son. Mike wheeled me down; then I was allowed to stand so I could scrub my hands and gown up before entering the unit. Mike gave me his arm and led me into the nursery. There was none of the coo or fuss of healthy babies, only the chirps of monitors, the hiss of ventilators, the ambient buzz of machines at work.

Mike put his arm behind his back, a signal for me to walk right behind him. *This place must be full of babies*, I remember thinking—it was a maze of incubators and cribs. Eventually Mike stopped and brought me to his side.

"Give me your hand," he said. I did, and he drew it forward, threading it through a plastic opening and a curl of tubing until I felt soft, flabby skin.

"That's his leg."

This is the part on TV where the music wells up, the camera goes hazy and I'm surrounded with a loving glow.

It wasn't so.

I needn't have worried about becoming attached. Once my hand was on Gus's leg, I was scared stiff. He was so connected up that I was sure I'd dislodge something, causing irreversible harm. Yet I kept my hand there; I didn't know what else to do with it.

"Is he awake?" I asked Mike. I felt no movement at all. A nurse heard me and came to talk to us. They'd given Gus a drug to paralyze him so he could be wired and intubated without hurting him too much. *Geez*, I thought, *he can't even feel me touching him*. I tried to picture him, but all I could think of was the scene in *ET* where the extraterrestrial is about to die.

The nurse explained that they were concerned about an opening between two of the chambers in Gus's heart, and about his lungs, which weren't completely developed. His fluids were out of whack and were being monitored as well; also his blood sugar levels, since he'd been born to a diabetic mother. Temporary paralysis left him unable to suck, so he was fed through an IV. There was more—she ticked off an inventory of other things they were monitoring—and when she finally told us that Gus had jaundice, I was almost relieved. Here was a medical term I'd heard before.

As usual, Mike asked pertinent questions: When would the doctor be in? When would the paralyzing medicine wear off? All through this I kept holding Gus's leg, patting it a little, forgetting he could feel nothing.

I was softening, but I still wasn't sure I wanted to spend a whole lot of time with Gus. That is, until the nurse left and I was able to hear Mike talking to him. First he asked me if it'd be OK for him to touch Gus for a while. "Yes! Sure!" I said, relieved to have him replace my hand with his.

"Hi Gus," I heard him say in the sweet soft voice that he saves for special moments. "Hi Gus," he said again. "How are you doin' today?" He called him Sweetie, told him he was a brave boy. It was beautiful to hear. This was finally the moment; I was melting with love and emotion—not for Gus, but for Mike. I wanted to keep visiting Gus just to hear Mike talk to him.

I felt Mike shift toward me. "How are you doing?" he asked. I let out a long breath. I was tired, I was sore. I hadn't stood up this long since before the Caesarean.

"We should get going," Mike said, then bid goodbye to Gus, using the same words I'd hear every day for the next month: "Fight the good fight, Gus."

Gus fought, but it was uphill all the way. No one seemed to know exactly what was wrong with him, what had caused the trauma at birth, or why he was continuing to struggle.

As the days wore on we did get flashes of good news, but it seemed that every good message was followed by something dire. The day they turned the jaundice lamps off was the day they discovered the simian creases in Gus's hands. The day the IV came out he had an X-ray that revealed he was missing a tailbone. One day a nurse dropped a pan in the nursery and Gus stirred. "He can hear!" she exclaimed, but when the doctors examined his ears, they found that the ear canals were oddly shaped and the ears themselves were set abnormally low on his head. Gus's head was big for his body, Dr. Ionnides told us one day. "But looking at you two," he chuckled, sizing up our skulls, "maybe it's just genetic." We acknowledged our melon heads and laughed long and hard—longer and harder than the remark merited, maybe, but what a relief in that tense and serious atmosphere.

Any of these things—the opening in the heart chamber, the simian creases, the lowered ears, the oversized head, the missing tailbone—could occur in an otherwise normal child. But the combination in one baby concerned Dr. Ionnides. When the genetic specialist from the University of Chicago came down for his monthly consult, Dr. Ionnides asked him to take a look at Gus. Again we got good news with the bad. The geneticist thought it unlikely that there was any genetic problem. The bad news? He wasn't *sure,* and so he ordered a full genetic workup. Another blood sample was taken from Gus's foot. Another two weeks of limbo. But almost immediately Gus started improving. And improving. And improving. This time there was no bad news coupled with the good. I'd been released from the hospital less than a week after Gus was born. With Mike working, the same friends who'd carted me to prenatal appointments now carted me to the hospital to see Gus. I was encouraged, no longer afraid we'd lose him. Mike and I both believed it was only a matter of time before we'd be at home with a normal little baby.

———   ———

Mike had been updating his family daily, and when his dad learned I needed help getting to and from the hospital, he drove the two hours from Lansing, a suburb south of Chicago, to stay with us. Grandpa qualified as immediate family, so he was allowed into intensive care. By this time we were able to take Gus out of his incubator and hold him a while. He was still tethered to machines, so cuddling was awkward; still, it was a pleasure to hold him, to sense what a bundle he was.

Mike's dad proved as gentle with Gus as Mike was, and I began to understand where Mike's tenderness had come from.

Mike and I visited Gus on our own after work. We'd take a break, then return for a few minutes around ten or eleven o'clock. It was on one of those late-night visits, during the fourth week, that a nurse greeted us with word that Gus could go home in a few days.

We each held him a long time that night, talking to him, telling him he'd be leaving with us soon. The next afternoon Mike had a job interview at the University of Illinois. The U of I was known for its great benefits plan, a factor becoming more critical to us by the day. Although I had good coverage under my disability benefits, Gus was covered under insurance from Mike's job. It had deductibles—we were responsible for 20 percent of Gus's hospital costs, which already exceeded $100,000. Soon we would be relying on credit cards to pay medical bills.

Mike came home at lunch for his suit and tie. I kissed him and wished him luck. As he left for the interview, his dad and I departed for the hospital.

We scrubbed, suited up in our gowns, and walked to Gus's bed, where a nurse laid him in our arms. Gus even took part of the bottle I fed him—already he was being seen by a speech therapist who taught us exercises that encouraged him to suck on the bottle. I'd been pumping breast milk since the day he was born, and we had quite a stash of it in Ziploc bags in the freezer.

Mike's father and I stayed a little longer than usual that day but finally left Gus alone to sleep. A nurse had told me earlier that Dr. Ionnides wanted to see me; I'd decided to wait until Mike was there. But the doctor spotted us in the hallway, called out, and quickly stepped over to grab my arm.

"Is your husband here?" he asked.

No, I said, he'd be coming later.

The doctor insisted on talking right away.

"Can Gus's grandpa come in?" I asked.

A flat No.

Dr. Ionnides was clearly nervous. "It'd been better if your husband were here . . ." he said. He led me clumsily to a chair in his office and closed the door.

"The genetic tests came back," he announced without preamble. "Gus has extra genetic material on his twelfth pair of chromosomes." His accent was a thick syrup; I understood the words but didn't immediately grasp their importance.

"That's good, right?" I asked, hoping against hope. Can't everybody use a little extra genetic material? "It'll make him even smarter, right?"

I knew Dr. Ionnides wasn't smiling.

"I'm afraid this is quite serious."

I started feeling nauseous. I could hear but couldn't comprehend. I caught some words: *rare, low IQ, genetic specialist, abnormal.* My head spun. I began to cry. Dr. Ionnides apologized. He said he wished he could have waited to tell me when my husband was there. He stood up, and I guessed he was waiting for me to stand, too, so I did. He led me back to Mike's dad and told me to have Mike call him with any questions.

When we got home, I went straight to bed. I was still there when Mike burst in a few hours later.

He was excited: the interview had gone well, Gus was about to come home, and all was right with the world. Then he saw my face. He climbed in bed and held me.

"What?" he said, "What is it? You have to tell me what's wrong."

Finally I was able to utter two words: "It's bad."

I cried some more. Mike held me, caressed me, told me I was all right, it would be all right. I concentrated and finally mustered a few more words.

"The genetic tests came back."

Mike didn't need to hear anything else.

Gus's official diagnosis was Trisomy 12p, which meant, as Dr. Ionnides had explained, that he had extra genetic material on the twelfth chromosome pair. How Gus came by it was a mystery. Mike and I were asked to give blood samples to see if either of us carried some sort of abnormality. It would be weeks before the results came back.

In the meantime, we'd been telling people that when Gus finally came home we'd have a big party. I wasn't so sure I could go through with it, but Mike was determined not to treat Gus's birth as a tragedy.

I had to agree. But while Gus's birth may not have been a tragedy, in my mind, his diagnosis certainly was. After all we did to make sure that baby was born healthy—lab visits and blood tests, strict diet and multiple insulin doses, doctor visits and appointments with specialists—we ended up with faulty goods. I had expected to feel triumphant, and instead I felt like a certified loser.

Gus arrived home on a Friday night, and we had his party the next day. It was a gorgeous fall day, much like the one three years

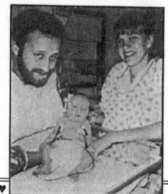

Gus 'n Us!

*Beth Finke and Mike Knezovich
announce the birth
of their son*

Gus Michael Knezovich

on September 3, 1986
weighing in at 8 lbs. 11 oz.

Gus will soon come to realize what we already know - that his birth and life are the product of loving and caring friends and family.
Thank you for the blood tests, phone calls, rides to the doctor, timely meals and snacks, encouragement and understanding throughout.

- Beth and Mike

☞ **NEW ADDRESS** ☜
604 West California, Urbana, IL 61801

Gus's birth announcement.

earlier when I first realized how much I loved Mike. Anne hung a "Welcome Home, Gus!" banner on the front of the house, where friends couldn't help but see it as they kept coming and coming with gifts and good wishes. Mike's sister, Kris, spent most of that day rocking Gus in our big old homemade rocking chair, singing and baby-talking to him. Gus was very content. On the surface, all seemed pleasantly normal.

But deep down in Gus's chromosomes, everything was abnormal. So, it seemed, were the gifts, the cards with "Congratulations—Babies Are Wonderful!" and this whole occasion. It was all fiercely bittersweet.

Yet Mike exuded a genuine sweetness. He carried Gus all over the house with him, often placing Gus's cheek next to his own and cooing to him. He inspected Gus frequently, made sure he was clean and comfortable, no rashes or anything. It was as if Mike had determined that his baby would never be in pain again.

My way of being with Gus was far less selfless. Doing things I wanted to do anyway, I incorporated Gus in ways that might look good to the slew of therapists who had been assigned to his case. I let the occupational therapist think our back-and-forth time on the porch swing was deliberately intended to stimulate Gus. With the piano back in our house, I sold my fiddle. (Neighbors must have cheered.) Earnings from the sale went toward paying a graduate student to teach me to play piano by ear; Gus lay across my lap as I practiced. And I let the speech therapist believe I was playing more now solely to improve his listening skills.

My former fiddle teacher recommended me to a local old-time string band that needed a piano player. "This is wonderful! Gus benefits so much from this!" his social worker complimented me. I had passed the audition, and she was sure I arranged for the band to practice at our house for Gus's sake. I nodded a response.

Snippets of time between diapering, feeding, burping, and bathing Gus were never long enough to do anything productive. They

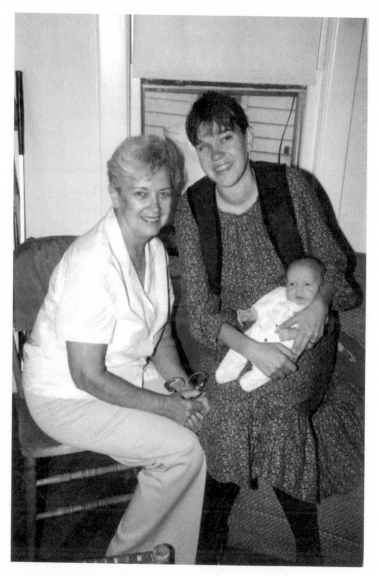

Flo (age seventy), Gus (age one month), and me (age twenty-seven; no eye prosthesis yet).

were long enough, however, to sit down and try out chord patterns from my lessons. I started experimenting with jazz, surprising my traditional string band with an occasional flat five or minor seventh. They tolerated it.

They tolerated a lot, actually. When I first joined, "Oh! Susanna" was the only old-time tune I knew. I brought my handheld tape recorder to every practice, listening at home to differentiate and memorize their repertoire. At gigs my memory would fail me; I had to be reminded what key to use for every tune. And instead of the traditional eye movement or foot kick to signify song endings, the lead musician yelled "Last time!" so that I could hear him over my playing.

I didn't know it, but practices and performances served as therapy. I would pound out chords when I was angry, play painfully slowly on melancholy days. Sequestered with a newborn, I practiced a lot. I improved but never achieved mastery. Blindness doesn't confer instant musical expertise.

Another myth says that hearing improves when sight is lost. In our case, it was Mike who heard Gus in the night, Mike who turned to me as we sat in the kitchen or living room and asked, "Is that Gus?"

As much as he loved his son, Mike wasn't immune to confusion and disappointment. Though I hadn't witnessed it, our friend Russ had seen Mike crying in the hospital bathroom shortly after the birth. Then one night, after Mike put Gus to bed, I became concerned that it was taking so long and finally went to check. I could hear the rhythmic creak of the rocker. I stood there. Mike was sobbing hard. When he could speak, he said simply, "I wanted to play baseball with him."

All that love and care given to Gus, and Mike would never receive the reward he had pictured. I wanted to pound my fists on the floor, scream, kick at a wall until I smashed a hole through it. But I did none of these things. Nor did I say anything. There was nothing to say.

When Gus had been home a couple of weeks, we were called to the university lab for the results of our genetic tests. We learned I had a "balanced genetic translocation"—two abnormalities that cancel out one another. They didn't affect me but caused the imbalance in Gus. In what Mike called "a bad cosmic joke," Gus's genetic problems had absolutely nothing to do with my being diabetic.

Maybe it was just the last straw, but this news hit me harder than anything else thus far. It was *my* fault. I couldn't do *anything* right.

It was probably the low point of my life. I cared for Gus day to day but struggled with my emotional burden. My initial coolness, when we'd thought we'd lose him, had given way to warmth until Dr. Ionnides gave his diagnosis. After that, I'd been angry at Gus. Now word of my own genetic abnormality was making me angry at myself, and that anger spilled all over Gus as well. He was *not* the child I had expected. All he'd done was bring more trouble.

So, yes, I did all the therapeutic exercises, I cuddled with him, I played the piano and spoke soft words to him. But none of it was heartfelt. Until one night, singing Gus to sleep, I started to cry. I was rocking in the chair Mike had occupied when he'd broken down. Gus lay across my lap. Suddenly, for no apparent reason, understanding washed over me: none of this was his doing. I had no earthly reason to blame him.

"You didn't want it to be like this," I said out loud to Gus through my tears. "It's not your fault, is it?" I gathered him into my arms and squeezed him to my shoulder where I could talk right into his ear.

"It's not your fault, Gus." Over and over I repeated it. I rocked and hugged him, finally able to love him and to tell him so.

5 | Another Sort of Trouble

We spent Labor Day 1989 at a picnic. I'd lain on a blanket with Gus; Mike played volleyball, fixed me a plate of food, visited with Anne while Billy tended the grill or changed the tap on the beer keg. It was a perfect day, the sun still summery enough to warm our skin, the air cool enough to hint that leaves would fall soon. We'd taken the tandem bicycle, with Gus behind us in a trailer.

Gus was asleep when we arrived home. I put him to bed, leaving Mike to put the tandem in the shed. It seemed to take him forever, and when I finally went to check, I found him on the porch steps, crying. I felt my way to his side and sat, squeezed his shoulder, asked what was wrong.

"I've got to tell you something, Beth," he said. He was deadly serious.

I braced myself. He had landed a good job—with benefits—at

the university. Had he been fired? Had one of our friends been diagnosed with a terminal disease? What a strange relief it was to hear the real reason for his misery.

"Anne? You mean *our* Anne?"

Mike's head nodded against my arm. Smiling, I squeezed his shoulder again.

"Of course you love Anne," I told him. "Who doesn't? I've been in love with her for years!" For over a decade, actually.

———

Back in 1977, my freshman year, Anne and I lived in the same residence hall. Long before we officially met, I knew who she was. A straight-A junior transfer student in graphic design, she was hard to miss—always surrounded by friends and always, always laughing. She wasn't petite by any means, but she was pretty, I thought, with chestnut hair to her shoulders, clear croissant-colored skin, and pleasant brown eyes.

During the 1978 spring semester Anne and I were assigned to the same dish room at our cafeteria jobs. After a few weeks of sharing small talk, I finally got up the nerve to stop at her dorm room one night.

"Hi!" she exclaimed. Her door had been wide open, of course. "C'mon in!"

She was hovering over a drawing table, a thin wooden stick in her hand. An art project, she explained. "You paint a white piece of paper black. Then, instead of drawing, you scratch."

Looking over her shoulder, I saw a whiskered old man emerging from the black page.

"When's it due?"

"Tomorrow."

"Aw, shoot. I was gonna ask if you wanted to join me for a beer."

"Sure!" she replied, setting down her pointed stick. She didn't stop to brush her hair or check the mirror or change clothes. She would finish the project later.

As expected, a night out with Anne was great fun. We went to the Illini Inn, the closest bar to our dorm. Anne knew almost everyone who walked in and introduced herself to the others. She lavished attention and affection on everyone. She stayed up late after we got home and still got an A on her drawing the next morning.

Anne and I maintained a casual acquaintance throughout college; not until after graduation, when our other friends departed, did we become close. We phoned each other most days, and Anne often surprised me with gifts, things she'd either made herself or picked up because they made her think of me. We met for breakfast once a week and had been meeting for happy hour each Friday until I began my weekly laser zaps in Chicago.

Unfazed by my worsening vision, Anne simply replaced the TGIFs with Wednesday evening get togethers. After the surgeries failed, we'd reverted to Fridays. She never complained about having to drive, and she matter-of-factly recited restaurant menus to me. She was perfectly happy to sit me at a table and fetch a pitcher for us. I didn't need to see perfectly to talk to Anne or listen to her wealth of stories. I didn't need to watch anything move, or move myself. With her I was contented, absorbed.

Now it sounded like Mike was feeling this way, too.

He started with New Orleans. Anne, Billy, Mike and I had spent a weekend in the French Quarter that spring. Anne was sneaking glances at him the whole time, he said. "And then on our last night there she gave me a kiss. More than just a friendly kiss. It flustered me at first, but then I sort of put it out of my head. Really, I was kind of flattered and I just wrote it off as innocent flirtation."

Absolutely, I thought. New Orleans, everyone knew, was a sexy place.

Mike went on, describing how unnerved he'd become when Anne flirted with him at his birthday party in June. He found himself enjoying it, he admitted. And now he was returning the attention, but fearing where it might lead.

Poor Mike. He'd fallen for Anne's enthusiasm, mistaken her caring and her attention for romance.

Feeling compelled to talk directly to Anne, Mike had asked her to lunch. "She about died. She said she was sorry for putting me in an awkward position. She just kept apologizing. By the time we were done, it was cool. She didn't seem embarrassed anymore. I told her I'd keep that conversation to myself."

Anne must have felt she should follow his lead. She and I were still getting together for weekly breakfasts and talking on the phone most days. There'd never been a whisper of this.

"I figured that was that," Mike said. "But at the picnic today, it flared up again."

Gus was due to start school the next day. We'd ordered him a wheelchair and built a ramp onto the house. With Gus occupied during weekdays, I planned on improving my Braille, walking more with the cane, getting back to my writing. This puppy love for Anne was something Mike would have to work through on his own.

"It's scary," he said.

I agreed. My fear had little to do with our marriage—he'd get over his crush, I was certain. I was more concerned about how his actions might affect our relationship to Anne. My blindness, and now Gus's problems, made it understandably difficult for some old friends to feel comfortable with us. Anne had stuck with me through all the surgeries. She'd put up with us after our apartment fire, come every day to do blood tests when I was pregnant. Anytime we needed a babysitter, she was there. Explanations were unnecessary. With Billy, too, things seemed comfortable. Mike's attitude improved on nights when we were out with them. Their friendship, especially mine with Anne, felt precious. I didn't want anything to screw it up.

I thanked Mike for his honesty, then suggested maybe we not see

Anne and Billy so much for a while. He agreed. I kissed him on the cheek and told him I was going to bed.

——— ——

Soon afterward, Mike announced he'd decided to train for a half-marathon scheduled for Memorial Day weekend, 1990. I was all for it. Since his confession an unspoken tension permeated our house, a quiet nervousness that we shared but never mentioned. The anxiety rushed out the door with Mike each day as he left to train, and I had begun to welcome my time without him.

The tension came back when he walked in the door. He snapped at me when I made simple mistakes in the kitchen or knocked into furniture while holding Gus. His outbursts were followed by exasperated sighs as he stomped out of the room.

One day I picked up the phone and begged Anne to come get me. "Bring Nancy if you want," I said. "I need to get *out* of here."

We met over lunch at Murphy's, a campustown joint where the three of us had hung out together as students. Anne and I had often met here with the British exchange students; it was the only place on campus that called itself a pub. Dim lights, solid dark wood tabletops with names carved into them.

"I'm worried about Mike," I announced as we ate.

"Why's that?" Nancy asked. Her voice sounded muffled. She must have been looking down at her food.

"He seems so tense all the time," I said, wiping the ketchup off my fingers. Seems I always end up with gooey stuff on my hands—I have to squeeze with one hand and use the other to guide and measure.

I waited for a response. Neither of them said a word. Maybe their mouths were full?

I asked Anne, "Haven't you noticed it when you and Mike go to play volleyball?"

Anne finished her bite. "No, I don't think so," she finally answered. "But we're just concentrating on volleyball."

I had put that team together years ago, when I could still see, and it continued in a park district league. Lately I'd been encouraging Mike to go out with the other players after the games; he'd become such a grouch that I really didn't want him around, and I thought maybe getting away from Gus and me on a regular basis would do him good. Mike and Anne alternated driving each week. Billy played occasionally, too, but skipped a lot of games because of work.

"Maybe Mike gets it out of his system by spiking the ball," Nancy offered.

"Maybe," I said, "but it sure doesn't last long. Maybe he should play volleyball every night. He screamed at me yesterday when all I did was drop a plate. It didn't even break!"

"Didn't his friend Julie at work just move away?" Anne suggested. "Maybe he's bummed about that."

I hadn't thought of that. He really did like Julie, and she'd moved to Minneapolis. Mike's best friend from kindergarten lived in Minneapolis, and Mike and I had visited up there before we got married. Mike loved it there, and the University of Minnesota was one of his top choices back when he was filling out law school applications. All this was before I'd lost my sight and law school was tossed out the window.

"Yeah, maybe that's it," I said.

Then we talked about Nancy's kids, about work. Anne and Nancy each offered to drive me home. I opted for Anne. After all those times leading me to the bathroom when we were out with Mike, Anne had become a very accomplished sighted guide. I felt almost as comfortable walking with her as I did with Mike.

Get-togethers like this confirmed my belief that Anne couldn't possibly be encouraging or reciprocating Mike's attentions. Our drives together provided plenty of opportunities for Anne to confess if she felt the need. Obviously, there was nothing to tell. Besides, no one could offer a blind friend an elbow at lunchtime and sneak off with the blind woman's husband that night.

During that autumn my sex life with Mike, which had suffered since Gus's birth, came to an end. Anne and Billy started working with a fertility specialist. Billy rarely played volleyball, worked even later hours, and rarely joined us for a night out. Mike's volleyball nights with Anne routinely lasted past midnight. Anne signed up for a weekly exercise class and started working out religiously at home. Friends complimented her new figure and new outfits: she was opting for short skirts and dresses now, a long way from the painter pants and sweatshirt ensembles of her college days.

At Christmas Billy announced he didn't want to bother with a tree. We both insisted Anne help us trim ours. It's a tradition with Mike and me to sip good wine while we decorate. We all enjoyed ourselves, Anne perhaps a little too much. She accepted Mike's offer to drive her the mile or two back to her house when the tree was finished. He was gone more than an hour.

I had to be an idiot not to know what was going on. I wanted to believe my friendship with Anne was important enough to make her reject Mike's advances. As long as I didn't ask her specifically about this, I could reassure myself.

It's grim living with someone who'd rather be elsewhere. I accepted every invitation to get out of the house, sometimes in preparation for the single life, other times just to escape Mike. I began using Gus as an excuse to stay home when Mike and Anne went out. It was no fun being with them anymore; their half-hearted attempts to make me feel welcome had become insulting.

Mike continued training for his half-marathon. On Memorial Day weekend, Anne offered to stand at the sidelines with me so I'd know when Mike reached the finish line. After the race, they naturally wanted to celebrate.

"You guys go ahead," I told them. "It's four o'clock. I'd better get home to relieve the babysitter." Anne asked if I was sure. Mike said he'd call around eight o'clock to see if Gus and I were all right.

While feeding and bathing Gus, I mentally ticked off the items from the Single Woman Checklist I'd been compiling in my head. I hadn't accomplished everything on that list yet, but I was close enough.

The phone finally rang at 9:30. I didn't answer.

Mike called many times after that—I didn't need caller ID to know who it was—but I just let it ring. I wanted him to worry.

He had plenty of reason to, really. Each ring of the phone was making me angrier, fueling my determination to escape him, escape Anne, escape this whole situation.

Mike was exhausted when he walked through our front door late that night. I didn't wait to hear his hello before I began shouting accusations. He didn't deny a thing. This horrible session seemed to go on for hours and hours. In the end, Mike admitted that he had been seeing Anne more than I knew. And for longer than I realized. During their encounters, he said, they couldn't keep their hands off each other. "I'm more in love with Anne than I was before," he confessed, beginning to cry, "and there's nothing I can do about it."

"Well, you can divorce me and marry Anne."

Blindness may have made me temporarily needy, but never so needy that I would tolerate living with someone who was that unhappy with me. I'd been blind for four years. The energy spent caring for myself left little for Mike. But now I was back. I imagined he and Anne had assumed divorce was not an option—"Because of Beth," you know. Now I was the one suggesting it.

Ironically, by suggesting the "D" word, I was actually helping Mike with a problem.

I slept on the couch that night. The next morning I slipped into the bedroom, found my special clipboard, and wrote: "I'll be back at four to get my things."

———

An Amtrak train stopped through town at 6:30 each evening. Two hours would be long enough to get ready. After collecting my wallet, insulin, and a few syringes, I snuck out the front door without waking Gus or Mike. I tapped my way to the bank. Funny thing, without needing my eyes to navigate, I could cry all I wanted.

After emptying my savings account, I headed for the university's swimming pool. I thought about where I'd go on the train. I knew my presence alone would be a challenge for whichever sister or friend I ended up with; that meant Gus would have to stay home with Mike. And with Anne, I guessed.

I'd almost reached the pool when a very familiar voice called to me from the street. "*Beth*. Will you get in the car? Please?"

I was tired of struggling with the damned cane. And Mike sounded like he needed more help than I did.

As Mike shifted into gear, he told me he'd seen Anne again that morning. He seemed wrung out. With everything else going on, I'd forgotten he'd run a thirteen-mile race the day before.

Anne had told Mike she loved him. But that she wouldn't leave Billy. "She said she didn't want to hurt him. Or you."

I was unimpressed. Hurting Billy and me is exactly what they'd been doing for months. The only thing stopping her now was that it was no longer a secret.

I twisted toward the back seat, felt for Gus's little feet and started tickling them.

"She said something about the consequences," he said, almost to himself. "Not a word about caring anything about Billy. Just 'The Consequences.' She is such a coward," he said, hitting the steering wheel and repeating "coward" over and over.

I have to admit, I didn't get it. But when we arrived home and Mike asked me to stay, I agreed. At least for one night.

I never left again. For the first week or two, I was simply too overwhelmed to make sensible arrangements. I didn't think we could fix our marriage, but I was too worn out to leave.

Mike seemed to want everything about his life to change. He quit his job and started a new one at the university. But his work all seemed trivial, compared to what was going on at home. After two weeks, he quit on the spot. He was miserable.

My routine at home changed, too. I had no desire to play the piano; instead, I listened to the stereo. Bonnie Raitt sang her bittersweet songs just for me. My blood sugars went on a roller coaster. I couldn't eat, which caused them to drop too low. Then anxiety caused stress, which drove them too high. I felt ill for weeks and was unable to differentiate between diabetic sickness and heartsickness.

I honed my independent living skills. And I decided if anyone had to leave our house, it would be Mike. I needed to live in familiar surroundings.

We discussed divorce, or at least separation. It felt good to say the words. If we could talk about splitting up, I figured, we could talk about anything.

——— ———

After that initial Memorial Day shock, followed by weeks of mourning for Anne and our old lives, we finally did start talking. Once we started, we talked, and talked, and talked. With Mike home and unemployed, we had nothing but time.

Mike admitted he wished he lived with someone who could see him, to compliment him when he looked good, to notice when he was tired or down. I told him I wished I lived with someone who liked traditional music and would be more supportive of my playing, and who would compliment me when the band sounded good.

Mike confessed he sometimes hated going out in public because of people's stares. I told him it was hard to be out by myself now—I'd sometimes get an odd sensation that Anne was watching me. Mike wanted to move away to some more interesting and exciting place; we probably would have by now, were it not for my blindness. Now the thought of moving daunted me. I wasn't sure I could learn to get around in a city I had never seen.

Mike never apologized for being frustrated with his life, with me, with our circumstances, or for falling in love with Anne. "But I'm sorry I was dishonest. And that I went through all that for a coward," finally explaining what he meant by this. The reason Anne didn't leave Billy, Mike had deduced, was that she was afraid of how it would look. As long as the affair was under wraps, she could maintain her identity as sweet, helpful, happy go lucky.

"Anne was a coward, and I was pathetic."

Mike had many theories about what had happened with us and Anne and our lives in general. I wasn't sure I agreed with all of them, but I listened. One thing we shared that summer was anger. At first Anne served as a good punching bag. But without her there to respond, the punches soon became unrewarding. By July we were more forthright in attacking each other.

Most of my friends had been Anne's friends, too. They were retreating, I'd often complain to Mike. "And it's all your fault."

"They weren't really your friends, and neither was Anne. Where were they when you were in the hospital? Did you guys ever actually talk about anything real? No. All the hard stuff fell to me."

He said he'd been so consumed taking care of me and Gus that he'd neglected old friendships. He blamed me for pushing Anne and Billy on him; he'd sunk so low that he couldn't recognize what small people they had been all along.

He said I was self-centered and arrogant, that I'd gotten caught up in all the attention lavished on me because of my blindness. I took him for granted. I was insensitive.

Painful as it was, talking—and arguing—brought us some relief. We'd been attracted to each other in the first place because of the way we thought, the way we could talk frankly. We hadn't done much of that in a long time.

We didn't know how or whether it made sense for us to stay married, but we decided to give it at least a summer. We vowed to keep talking, to discover whether we liked who our partner had become.

By the end of August neither of us had contacted a lawyer. We hadn't yet discussed custody issues. Still, Mike and I often wondered aloud if we might be better off going our separate ways.

——— ———

Whatever we eventually decided, I knew I needed to work on becoming less arrogant and more independent.

You might not think arrogance would result from a new disability. Self-doubt, even self-hatred? Perhaps. But ever since I'd lost my sight, people had told me how wonderful I was, had applauded me for even the smallest accomplishments. I was praised for buckling my own seat belt, applauded for tying Gus's shoes, revered for washing the dishes. Hardly a day passed without someone telling me I was smart, courageous, or even inspirational. And because losing my sight and bearing a severely handicapped child hadn't killed me (nor had I killed myself), I felt immortal. I was convinced that my crises had left me with wisdom that made me superior to those around me.

It was an odd assortment of feelings to lug around. I could be unsure of myself when pouring hot water for tea or matching Gus's socks, but at the same time oddly invincible. The self-confidence that had served me well when I was first coping with blindness had gradually morphed into ugly arrogance.

My haughtiness, I came to realize, had helped dismantle my friendship with Anne, providing her with a rationale for the affair.

She'd witnessed my behavior toward others, especially Mike. While she was living with a man who doted more on his co-workers than on her, she saw in my husband a man who bent over backward to care for me, a man who loved his son no matter what. She'd watch Mike. Then she'd look at me, carrying on as if Mike wanted nothing more than to do the Blind Wonder Girl's bidding. She noted how seldom I thanked Mike for his help. She knew he deserved better treatment, and she was prepared to offer it.

Haughtiness had also prevented me from acknowledging early signs of an affair. In fact, Mike had told me everything I needed to know on the night of the Labor Day picnic. I hadn't heard his cry for help. I thought so highly of myself that I couldn't imagine anyone, let alone Anne and Mike, willfully hurting me.

In the end, it didn't take much work to lose the arrogance—the affair was quite humbling. Developing independence was a tougher problem. Using my white cane, I walked to the bank and took over our checking account. With the help of a teller and my hand-held cassette player, I recorded the check numbers and the amounts of checks cashed in the past month, then calculated the balance.

My volunteer reader that year was an accountancy major. She was delighted to huddle around my talking computer with me each week, to read bills aloud and listen as I keyed in the information. Soon I was in charge of paying the bills, figuring out the budget, and depositing checks. It pleased me to take charge of these tasks again.

In the fall I passed the probationary period at a job I'd started midsummer. I was gaining more responsibility, more money, and, best of all, more respect. I made new friends at work, people who didn't know Anne, Billy, or Mike. Mike wasn't terribly interested in socializing with these new people, which was fine with me. I liked it that he was known at work only as that friendly guy who drove me to work sometimes.

Mike and I made other changes. We visited Minneapolis and toyed with the idea of moving there. I became more determined to lighten Mike's load, to help him feel less responsible for everything in our lives. I worked hard at sharpening my skills and I filled out applications for guide-dog schools. If we stayed together, a guide dog would help our marriage; if not, I'd definitely need a dog anyway.

The more I did on my own, and the more independent I felt, the more confused I was about my life with Mike. Why work so hard to stay married? Even after our long hard summer, things *still* weren't right between us. He still snapped sometimes; just being in his presence often left me a bundle of nerves. And I wasn't sure I could trust him.

—————

In November Mike cashed in the retirement money he'd received when he left his university job. After paying off some bills, he suggested we splurge on a hotel in Chicago. We couldn't afford it; it'd be hard to find a sitter for Gus; I wasn't sure I wanted to spend all that time alone with Mike. But his enthusiasm was so refreshing that I succumbed.

We started the weekend at Andy's, a joint I'd enjoyed on an escape from Braille Jail. Not a fancy spot, but it has good live jazz. Mike grabbed a *Chicago Reader* from the stack by the door. We sat at the bar, ordered beers, and Mike flipped through the paper, reading out bands and clubs the two of us might enjoy. It was fun to be among city people, to act like we belonged there. We picked out a blues club for later and headed back to the hotel to get ready for dinner. I counted the dings in the elevator and proudly announced when we'd arrived at our floor. Mike led me to our room. We still had hours before we needed to leave. The pillows were fluffed, the sheets crisp. Slipping between the covers with Mike, I tried not to think about Anne.

Later we set off for a restaurant that a friend had recommended. I had asked for a place that would be truly Chicago, with no tourists or suburban kids. This fit the bill. Unfortunately, it also seemed to have no waitresses. The restaurant was lit up, Mike said, and the front door unlocked, but we were the only ones there. We might have found it romantic, but waiting so long for menus began to make us antsy.

The situation was typical at that time. I often felt under pressure to make things work out; the smallest detail seemed critical. As we waited, the now familiar nervousness crept over me. Mike had listed off restaurants from the *Reader,* but I had argued for my friend's suggestion.

Mike and I often had conflicts over traveling. I always liked to go where I knew people, liked to get recommendations from insiders on what to see and do. Mike prefers adventure, the unknown. When things turn out for the good, he feels truly rewarded.

I had persevered on this night, and it was looking like we weren't even going to eat.

We were both quiet. I could smell spaghetti sauce or garlic bread somewhere. The tablecloths were vinyl, and I pictured one of those squat glass candle holders encased in plastic netting. This wasn't a cool city place. It was just a Midwestern Italian restaurant.

The waitress finally arrived and brought us some wine. It was good. We ordered. She brought the food. It was bad. At least I think it was bad—I took a few bites, but I just couldn't eat. I was so disappointed. We'd had such a nice time at Andy's, laying out our choices for this evening. I'd actually started thinking maybe Mike, Gus, and I could leave Urbana together, maybe for Chicago. I'd even felt at ease in that fancy hotel.

But then we ended up *here.* And it was my idea. Things seemed to be going this way for Mike and me all the time now: we'd feel upbeat, and then something bad would happen to bring things crashing down around us. It was exhausting. I wondered if we should finally give up.

"Mike?" I said, interrupting a long silence. "I need to ask you something."

His mouth was full of mediocre spaghetti. "What?" he finally asked.

"Do you want to get a divorce?"

He was quiet again. "You know, I've been giving it some thought."

I started playing with my fingernails, waiting. It was a habit I'd developed, rubbing each fingernail with the fingertips of my other hand, to check if there were any funny ridges. Flo always said you know you're healthy if your fingernails are firm and straight.

"Stop doing that!" Mike ordered, grabbing both my hands under the table, holding onto them. "And no, I don't want a divorce."

I raised my head so he could see my eyes, which were filling with tears.

"I love you, Beth. You know that, don't you?" He was still squeezing my hands under the table. I couldn't say anything. "It's been awful, I know."

"I didn't think it was going to be *this* hard," I responded while laughing, sort of. It was that kind of laugh you laugh when really you're crying. Snot flew out of my nose. I pulled my hands away from Mike's to find a paper napkin.

"Well, *I* knew it was going to be this hard, but it's going to get better. Don't you think it's already better than it was?"

"Yeah, I guess so. I mean, look at us. You're mad we're at this restaurant, and I'm bawling." I laughed again, producing more snot. Mike shoved his napkin into my hand. I rubbed my face again and continued.

"You don't think you'd have a better life with someone else?"

"I don't *want* to be with someone else," Mike answered, sounding exasperated now. "I thought for a while I might. Our lives seemed so screwed up. I'd see people in their minivans, you know, with baby seats in the back, and I'd think, 'Gee, that would be good, that kind of life.' But Beth, you know me, I'd *never* want that."

He was right. I just couldn't picture it.

"Just goes to show: the minivan with a doting wife and mother behind the wheel looked good to me. I could go to work every day, come home, dinner would be ready. I'd play with the kids a little afterward and the wife would put them to bed. I wouldn't have to talk to her much because she wouldn't understand what I was doing at work—she'd be so involved with the kids, you know. I'd do all my thinking and talking at work, she'd take care of the house and kids, and then I'd take her to the company Christmas party. Oh, and I'd golf on weekends."

"That doesn't sound so good now?"

Mike squeezed my hands so hard they almost hurt. "I don't want *that*! That's what I'm trying to tell you. Things just got so bad, I got brainwashed."

He kept raising and lowering his hands for emphasis; mine rose and fell with them.

"I love you, Beth. You know that, don't you?" he repeated.

Until that moment, I hadn't been sure. Now I found myself trusting his words again. It felt like that magical day in our Urbana kitchen years ago, or like when he stuck his hand into Gus's incubator and told him to fight the good fight.

"Yes," I said, squeezing back, "I do."

He came around the table, turned my face toward his, and gave me a big kiss. Feeling for his ear, I whispered, "I love you, too."

Back home, Gus continued attending school. I made some money working part-time and performing gigs with the band. Mike sent out résumés to employers in Champaign-Urbana and Minneapolis. He used some spare time to take a class at a community radio station, qualified for a broadcast license, and became a volunteer "air shifter" with his own weekly morning show. Gus and I were Mike's biggest fans, joining him in the studio for his first fundraising drive. By then I had taught myself the accordion (something to play at my band's outdoor gigs), and I brought it along. "Please pledge," Mike begged his listeners. "If you don't, Beth's gonna play that thing." Gus cooed in the background, the phone rang and rang, and Mike met his pledge goal.

Before Christmas, Mike accepted a consulting position with a small startup software company. Spyglass was founded in 1989, when a couple of whizzes from the University of Illinois engineered new data-visualization software; they soon teamed up with some business types. Group health insurance was too expensive for tiny Spyglass to offer its employees. The owners themselves were mostly living off savings and credit cards.

Eventually they attracted investors, hired an experienced business person, and offered Mike a salaried position. He became invigorated by the buzz surrounding a growing software firm in the 1990s. Night after night he'd come home brimming with stories about what he'd learned that day, who he'd met. Some nights, too, he'd come home with pieces of paper rewarding good work.

"If this company makes it," he told me, explaining what stock options were, "these will be worth something."

6 | Pandora

I never really liked dogs much. I was afraid of them, actually. I had no idea what was involved in taking care of a dog—we'd never had pets when I was a child—but it seemed like a lot of extra work. So the idea of a guide dog never appealed to me.

But then I had two problems in one month, both on the same stretch of busy road. Once, walking along the sidewalk, I inadvertently veered down a driveway and into the street. The other time I had an insulin reaction while I was walking, so I never quite learned how I ended up in the middle of that same busy street.

And so, taking one more step toward my goal of independent living, I investigated guide dog schools and applied to two: one was in California, the other in New Jersey. Mike jokingly referred to the latter as the "Harvard of guide dog schools," but he was serious about his preference for it. The Seeing Eye had the longest tradition, having pioneered the guide dog concept in the United States. Me? Since I might be there during winter, I fancied the California sunshine. In truth, I was impressed by both.

Competence with a white cane is a prerequisite for any guide-dog program. My skills, though rough around the edges, were adequate. But there were other factors: Did I have children? Did I work? Did I use public transportation? Some questions were intended to help match a student with the right dog. Others were to determine whether *I* was a good candidate for a dog.

During my interviews I expressed my ambivalence about dogs, and my candor concerned the school in California enough that they were reluctant to accept me. Not so with The Seeing Eye, so my decision became academic. In January 1991 (just at the time of the Gulf War) I headed off to Morristown, New Jersey.

——— ———

Besides my doubts about owning a dog, I had doubts about leaving Mike. Things were going well for us; we seemed to be talking honestly with each other now, enjoying each other more. He gave me no reason to mistrust him. Still, I worried that my four-week absence might lead him into temptation. The thought of leaving Mike to live in a dorm with a bunch of blind people also evoked memories of Braille Jail. I did my best to fight off worries, concentrating instead on arranging babysitters for Gus and packing for my month away.

From the start, The Seeing Eye was the antithesis of Braille Jail. Once accepted, I was expected to pay for my dog. Some schools retain ownership, but when you leave The Seeing Eye, your dog is *yours*. To reinforce the concept of ownership and responsibility, The Seeing Eye asked me for $150. It had to be my money. (I couldn't, for example, get the local Lions Club to donate on my behalf.) I could pay in installments, but one way or another, I had to come up with the $150.

It was the biggest bargain of my life. In addition to providing nearly a month of in-residence training with a specially bred dog, The Seeing Eye also provided round-trip airline tickets from Champaign and had a driver waiting when I arrived in New Jersey.

At the school I was immediately introduced to Miss Early, who, over the past several months, had been training a dog for me. (I learned later that my dog was born at The Seeing Eye, lived there with her mother for six weeks, and then went to a family who had volunteered to raise her until she was a year old.) Next I met Gloria, the nurse, who showed me the hallway refrigerator where I could find juice for low blood-sugar episodes. She taught me the short route from my dorm room to her office, which was staffed twenty-four hours a day.

"Do you always put the diabetics right next to the nurse's office?"

"You bet," she replied. Since diabetes is the leading cause of blindness in adults, they were quite familiar with the disease.

"You'll be in here a lot," Gloria continued. "We'll keep your insulin here, plus there are four blood-sugar tests a day and nightly foot inspections." Diabetics are notorious for having troublesome cuts and sores on their feet, and the nursing staff wanted to be sure that all the walking we did with the dogs didn't cause foot problems. I'd never had daily inspections before, even during hospital stays. These people were serious about diabetes. I liked that.

In fact, they were serious about everything. After dinner the first night, we all piled into an upstairs meeting room. Since most of the students were replacing dogs and hadn't used their canes for years, it was a clumsy migration. The first lecture was actually kind of a pep rally. We were introduced to the staff, who told us what a great bunch of dogs they had for us—we'd meet them the next afternoon. Next we were given leashes, chain collars, and two brushes and a comb for the dog's grooming. The return students ("retreads," as they were known) were then dismissed. The three other first-timers and I stayed, learning to put on and remove a harness. Even on a stuffed "dummy" dog, this simple exercise seemed daunting. *This, I thought, is going to be a lot of work.*

On the first morning, we were given the luxury of sleeping in until seven o'clock. "Don't get used to this," one trainer warned. "Once you have your dogs, you'll be getting up *much* earlier for park time." (Park time meant taking the dogs outside.) He was right: between park times, meals, field training, and lectures, our days ran from 5:30 A.M. to 8:00 P.M.

As we finished breakfast that first morning, Miss Early reminded our group that she would introduce us to our dogs that afternoon. "I'll come and get you one at a time. Have your leashes ready."

She asked if we had any questions. No one did, or at least no one said anything.

"Remember, there is no such thing as a stupid question. Now, are you sure none of you has a question? Not just about getting your dogs. I mean, questions about anything going on here?"

"Well, yes," I said, suddenly feeling an overwhelming urge to challenge that no-such-thing-as-a-stupid-question proclamation. "I have a question."

"Ms. Finke?"

"Yeah, that's it," I said. "Why do we all have to go by our last names?"

"It's tradition. When they first started training dogs for the blind here long ago, no one really respected blind people. The folks who started The Seeing Eye thought using formal names was one way to show respect."

"So do I have to refer to my fellow students by their last names all the time?"

"Really, you can use whatever names you want. But the trainers will always address you formally, and you're required to use our formal names, too."

"And the dress code?" Women were required to wear dresses and men jackets at lunch. I didn't mind—I actually *like* wearing dresses and skirts—but I was curious. "It's the same philosophy?"

"Partly, but mainly it's because most of our tour groups come through during lunchtime."

"So they just want us to look good for the tour groups?" I asked, a little miffed.

"It's more that we often have corporate types visiting at lunch. There's always a chance that they might need to hire someone for a job someday; you never know. We want you to look good, just in case."

We also learned that, while German shepherds were once the breed of choice, their tendency toward relatively early hip dysplasia has led trainers to add other breeds that can have longer, more active careers.

That afternoon I met my dog. I heard a jingle-jingle-jingle coming from the direction of the lounge. I made my way toward it with my cane.

"Here," Miss Early said, patting a chair cushion, "sit down." I sat. "Now say, 'Pandora, come!'"

I did, and Pandora came to me. I had absolutely no idea what to do. Miss Early showed me how to attach a leash to Pandora's collar, then instructed me to pet my dog.

My dog.

"We won't be using harnesses until tomorrow," Miss Early explained. "Today is a day for you and Pandora to have fun, to get to know each other."

Pandora seemed nice enough; she didn't jump on me or growl or sniff my crotch. She was a black Labrador retriever, I was told. Miss Early led us back to my room, and Dora and I spent our first day together.

———

The next morning Pandora and I were part of the first group to work after breakfast. (Diabetics always worked right after eating, to prevent low blood sugar reactions.) I figured we'd stay on The Seeing Eye's grounds. Instead, a van transported us to the middle of Morristown where there were sidewalks and street corners, railroad crossings and stoplights. It was scary.

My first lesson, of course, involved getting Pandora into the van. "Tell her to sit and rest there by the door," Miss Early instructed. "You get in first and sit down, always keeping your hand on her leash."

Once I was seated Miss Early asked me to call Pandora.

"Pandora!" I called toward the open door, "Come!"

Pandora immediately jumped into the van and sat at my feet. After two other students followed the same routine, Miss Early got in and started the van. Pandora scooted forward and sat next to her. She didn't say anything about this, so neither did I.

Before long Pandora and I were standing on a Morristown sidewalk. I was visited by a familiar sense of disappointment. *I'm not trying hard enough to think positively. The other students are excited; I'm just worried.* It reminded me of meeting Gus: here was another made-for-TV moment, unrealized. This time I was supposed to be enraptured by and feel complete trust in my Seeing Eye dog. But I had too many doubts to let any magic materialize.

I still couldn't see a damned thing and here I was, about to walk down a completely unfamiliar street. This dog I'd just met was supposed to keep me from harm.

Miss Early stood slightly behind me at my right. "OK," she instructed, "tell her to go forward."

I never had a chance. The minute Pandora heard the "f" word, she bolted toward the next curb as I held on for dear life.

"Don't grip her harness so tightly! Stay loose!"

Stay loose? At this speed? This was the fastest I'd walked down a sidewalk without a sighted guide.

"And stand up straight! C'mon, straight! That's better."

My mother would have loved Miss Early.

"Now concentrate!"

I'd been thinking about my posture and forgot for a second that I was negotiating a sidewalk. It was amazing, really. I hadn't been able to lose myself in thought for even a moment while walking with a white cane. And, like many blind people, I had developed a defensive crouch. Now I strode like a model on a runway.

"Talk to your dog."

Yeesh. Concentrate *and* hold onto the harness *and* stand up straight *and* talk to the dog?

Suddenly she warned me that there was a car parked across the sidewalk ahead of us. Just as suddenly I forgot about staying loose, squeezing the harness as we approached it. Miss Early guided Pandora and me around the car—I could tell from her tone that she shared my exasperation about cars blocking sidewalks. Learning to negotiate such obstacles was for later lessons.

She kept reminding me to stay focused and to keep talking to my dog. I would concentrate for a few moments, then drift off in worry; remind myself to loosen up; notice I was slouching, then straighten. Gradually I began to pay better attention to my left hand grasping the harness. I could feel Pandora's gait. In the middle of all this, a grin had planted itself on my face. Walking with Pandora was a delight.

I turned to smile at Miss Early. I bet she cracked a smile herself.

It was a great beginning, but the hard work lay ahead. Every minute of every day at The Seeing Eye, I was leashed to Pandora. At night she was chained to my bedpost. Every weekday I followed the same schedule: up at daybreak; feed, water, and "park" Pandora; go to the nurse's office for a blood test and insulin; then breakfast at my assigned seat. After breakfast, we boarded the van with our trainer; then back to The Seeing Eye for midmorning tea break. Before lunch we groomed the dogs and put them through an obedience ritual.

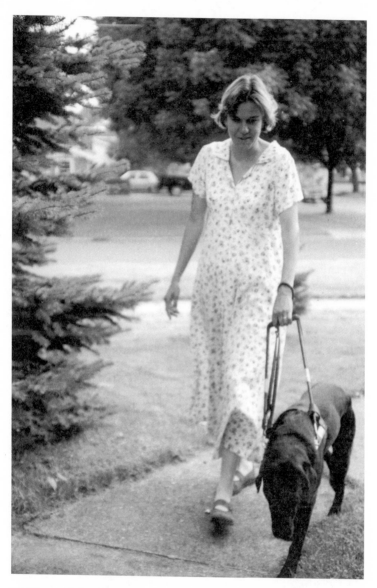

Walking with Pandora.

Despite our auspicious first trip, I began to have problems with Pandora. She still seemed more attached to Miss Early.

"She's used to the way I talk," Miss Early told me after I complained about Pandora not responding to my "Forward!" command. "But don't worry, she'll get used to your voice."

To be fair, I was as foreign to Pandora as she was to me. Every time we stopped at a curb, I'd be the first to step down. "Don't get ahead of your dog!" Miss Early had to keep telling me. "Remember: she leads *you*."

Things did improve, and day by day I warmed to Pandora. Then we hit a wall. After our first solo trip, during which Miss Early observed us from afar rather than tagging immediately behind, Dora turned stubborn. It was almost as if someone had switched dogs on me during the night. She started lunging at other dogs as we worked. She balked during our daily obedience routine. Worst of all, she stopped for no reason in the middle of a walk.

Once, after just such an instance, I corrected her and got her rolling again. Miss Early called out "Keep her going! Keep her going!"

"F—k you!" I snapped. "I'm doing everything I can!"

Suddenly Pandora stopped. Not realizing why, I told her she was bad and tried to yank her ahead. Then I discovered that she'd stopped for a curb. I had done exactly the wrong thing.

The next night I broke down crying during dinner. The students at my table were going on and on about how great their dogs were. I was envious. I worried that Pandora didn't like me. I was sorry about swearing at Miss Early. And I was sure that I was a bad dog handler.

As I fought back tears, it dawned on me that no one sitting around me could see. Why hold back? They wouldn't even know or care. This notion made me even more miserable. As I left the dining room, Miss Early said something to me, and I started blubbering. Pandora kept walking as though nothing was amiss. Another trainer, Mr. Frank, called out. "Ms. Finke! Anything wrong?"

I stopped. "Not really."

He caught up to me and grabbed my free arm. He was looking me right in the eyes, I could tell. Tears were streaming down my face. "Well, you know, there's something about the way you look," he said. "I've been here a long time, and I can tell—"

I choked out a laugh. He guided me toward my room. I sat on my bed; he sat across from me, on my roommate's bed, and handed me a Kleenex.

"Did anything unusual happen today?"

I told him about my trials with Pandora. Today had gone no better than the previous day, when I'd had my little tantrum. Today Pandora had frozen when we encountered a construction zone; Miss Early had to bail us out.

"I must be doing something wrong," I mumbled, more to myself than to him. He shoved another Kleenex into my hand. We were both quiet for a while.

"I guess I feel some pressure for Pandora to work out. That lecture the other night . . . it made me realize how much trouble goes into training the dogs."

"Ha! Our brainwashing works!" he laughed. Then his voice took a serious tone.

"Look, this week is an especially difficult one. The dogs lose all their motivation. They used to work for their trainer but now the trainer's not around so much. All the dogs are like this right now. They're looking at you guys and thinking, 'Why should I do this *for them*?'"

I nodded.

"Keep praising her when she does well. You're the one who feeds her, you groom her, you're with her day and night. She'll love working for you. You'll see."

"I hope you're right," I murmured, still wiping my eyes. "I mean, it all makes sense." Again there was a quiet time.

"Is there anything else going on that you want to talk about? Are you homesick, maybe?"

I thought about it. "Thanks, no," I said finally, giving him permission to leave.

——— ———

I hadn't been phoning Mike every night the way I had from Braille Jail. For one thing, I didn't have the time. For another, Mike wasn't worried, so I didn't feel compelled to let him know I was OK. When we did connect, Mike always seemed curious and encouraging, asking lots of questions about what Pandora and I were doing. He listened intently to my answers and even helped with problems sometimes.

"They want me to talk to her all the time," I complained once. "What am I supposed to say to her? She's a dog!"

"You always talk to Gus," Mike suggested. "Just pretend you're talking to him."

It was a great idea, and it worked. Mike's encouragement over the phone made me feel good. What I was doing interested him, and he wanted to share my experience as best he could. We seemed like partners again. I was growing more hopeful about our future together.

Before I left for New Jersey, Mike and I had discussed the idea of a visit. During one of our calls he brought it up again.

"That'd be great, but it's crazy, really," I said.

"I know, it's expensive, but your brother lives pretty close to Morristown. I could stay at his place. Then there'd be just the cost of the flight. And I can find someone to take care of Gus."

I wasn't thinking of money—I'd forgotten about money altogether, as I had no use for it at The Seeing Eye.

"We'd only be able to see each other during visiting hours." In addition to the formal names and dress codes, The Seeing Eye limited visits to specified hours. "And you can't come to my room." We could only meet in a public space—the lounge, the grounds. No conjugal visits.

"Wow, they *are* conservative."

"They say it's a privacy issue. They don't let anyone in the dorm rooms except students and staff. Not even when they give tours."

"You know, I like that."

I liked it, too. It seemed consistent with the whole approach.

"I want to see this place, Beth. And I want to meet Pandora. And I want to see you. I miss you."

So midway through my training, Mike and my brother, Doug, paid me and Pandora a visit. They checked in at the front desk, and Pandora and I met them in the lounge. I had to remind both of them not to call Pandora by name. "You can call her anything else," I said, suggesting names like Spike or Rover or Ribsy. "Just don't call her by her real name when she's in harness. It could distract her from her work—she might be tempted to look your way instead of paying attention to where we're going."

It was like an old-fashioned date. I walked proudly as Dora and I led Mike and Doug around the grounds, giving them the lowdown. Our time together was too brief, but it was a nice interlude.

———

Once the retreads had gone, Pandora and I received a week of intense individual attention. We went to a grocery store and a hospital. We even took a train ride so Pandora would know how to help me get on and off safely. Long-time residents of Morristown are completely accustomed to encountering Seeing Eye dogs—especially with the trainers, who travel around town with each dog much longer than its future blind owner does.

If Miss Early held my outburst against me, she never let on, remaining the consummate professional. And Dora improved. She excelled on a trip through a shopping mall, and passed with flying colors one of our final tests: guiding me through a gauntlet of other dogs let loose from The Seeing Eye breeding kennel.

Even more important, she managed "intelligent disobedience." On one of our trips a Seeing Eye van turned right on red in front of us, just after I'd told Dora to go forward at a green light. Pandora spotted the approaching van and refused my command. This is one of the more difficult and critical tasks for a guide dog.

I was excited to return home with Pandora when the day arrived, but full of nerves, too. I was still packing, unpacking, and repacking when Miss Early knocked on our door to say it was time. We were uncharacteristically quiet during the van ride to the airport. After showing me how to get through security with Pandora, Miss Early walked us onto the plane. She told Pandora to sit, then shoved Pandora's butt under the seat in front of me. Pandora somehow fit comfortably there, her head resting between my feet. Miss Early gave me a hug, said a tearful goodbye to Pandora, and we were off.

7 Adventures with Gus

From the day he was born, the quality and availability of services for Gus were much better than they'd been for me. While he was still in intensive care—even before we knew about his genetic problem—the hospital contacted the local agency that serves kids with developmental disabilities. His traumatic birth, coupled with my blindness, suggested that we might need extra help. The Developmental Services Center immediately enrolled Gus in their program for children ages zero to three. There would eventually be plenty of paperwork, but it was treated as a formality, not a prerequisite. With Gus, it always seemed to be act first, ask questions later.

He was evaluated by specialists and offered a smorgasbord of services. He was seen—regularly, and in our home—by physical, occupational, and speech therapists, and even an adaptive-toy specialist. A state agency made referrals to medical specialists. For those who qualified, as we did, it also footed doctor's bills and covered special equipment. Again, there was paperwork, and we took the appointments as they were available, but someone always assumed an active role in helping us.

Though multiple entities were involved, everyone seemed to know the drill and things got done. Gus's neurologist, for instance, had worked with all these agencies before; he knew the terminology and was diligent about crossing t's and dotting i's exactly as the bureaucracies required.

Mike and I no doubt affected how things went for Gus, too. We were battle tested by now, more assertive than when I was newly blind, more apt to trust our own instincts and to question authority. At one point, for example, a specialist determined that Gus was hydrocephalic: extra fluid in his skull was creating pressure that prevented his soft spot from hardening. Our doctor explained that a shunt (basically a drainage tube) could be surgically implanted to relieve the pressure. So we saw a neurosurgeon. This was one of the oddest appointments we ever had. Upon looking at the CT scan and X-rays, he declared that Gus had only half a brain.

Gus's neurologist was as dumbfounded by the surgeon's finding as we had been. He essentially counseled us to disregard it. We did so, happily. To this day the encounter remains a mystery. But we were still left with a decision about the shunt. Apart from the fact that it required major surgery, having a shunt would present ongoing problems and demand more special care for Gus.

Years before, we both might simply have said, "OK." But we discussed it and Mike asked the doctor whether there were any medical alternatives. We learned that, in some cases, simply using a diuretic could solve the problem. The odds were against it, but we decided to give it a try.

It worked. No surgery.

Then there was the pediatric ophthalmologist in Chicago. Actually, there were two. We were referred to a doctor experienced with kids who had special problems. Her resident conducted the preliminary exam. He looked at Gus's eyes, saying nothing to us about what he saw. Anxiety grew—I can't tell what's going on if people don't tell me, plus my history with medical events had me expecting the worst.

When he finally spoke, he seemed more interested in Gus's genetics than his eyes, asking question after question. We told him about my balanced translocation, and he asked whether the rest of my family had been tested for it. In fact, our geneticist had written a letter explaining the situation and how to get tested, and we had sent a copy to everyone in my family. What they did with that information was their business.

We told the resident all this. He asked whether any had been screened. "It's Russian Roulette if they don't."

I didn't much like this interrogation, mostly because I was eager to find out about Gus's eyes. Mike was stone quiet. I later learned that he didn't appreciate the young doctor equating Gus's existence with a losing round of Russian Roulette.

The senior physician concerned herself only with Gus's eyes. We learned they were fine mechanically, but there was no way to tell how optical information was reaching his brain, or how he was processing it. On balance, it was pretty good news.

Before we left, Mike politely detailed the resident's behavior and made clear that it was unacceptable to us, wondering aloud whether the resident was fit to practice medicine. The doctor listened and apologized for her charge's behavior. What came of that, I don't know, but the exchange marked how differently we had come to approach the system and its authorities.

———

It was hard keeping up with all of Gus's appointments, but I tried. We put a huge calendar up in the hallway; I festooned it with Braille notes on sticky labels. This worked well most of the time, though there were occasional mistakes. Most appointments involved home visits, so it didn't much matter if I messed up; people just appeared. But it was unnerving to be surprised, especially by the public health nurse or the social worker.

The public health nurse was always on the lookout for unsanitary conditions. I'm a slob, always have been, always will be. It has little to do with my blindness, but I'm sure the public health nurse had her own thoughts on that.

Gus's first social worker nosed about for a different sort of dirt. How were things between Mike and me? Good, I told her. And in fact at the time they *were* good, but she didn't believe me. We were off schedule: according to what her textbooks said about parents of disabled infants, we should be having marital conflicts by now. She pried and prodded, suggesting at each visit that we had problems I'd never before considered. She nagged us to join a parent support group she was facilitating. When it finally became clear that I wasn't in the market for whatever she was selling, she told me I was in denial.

It spoiled my entire day. I racked my brain—Could it be true? Was I in denial?

"What's wrong?" Mike asked the minute he arrived home. It killed me the way he could look at my face and instantly know something was up. "Are you OK? Is Gus sick?"

"We're both fine. The social worker was here today."

"I wish you wouldn't see her anymore." Mike picked Gus up from his baby seat and made kissy noises on his cheek.

"We have to if we want to get all the services for Gus."

"You don't need no stinking social worker, do you Gus?" Mike said in his best movie tough-guy voice.

But a lot was at stake, including physical therapy and speech therapy. I was setting the table as we talked. We were having baked pork chops with sauerkraut. When I cooked, I used only the oven, still not trusting what I'd learned in Braille Jail about skillets and stovetops.

"Of course he needs those things, but I don't understand why she has to come to our house all the time."

Mike rarely had to deal with the social worker directly, but he never escaped my mood afterward.

"So what did she say today?"

"That I was in denial about Gus."

"F—k!"

I laughed. That was exactly what I had wanted to say all afternoon. I had let her plunge me into this funk of self-doubt. Suddenly it seemed absurd to have spent my whole afternoon down in the dumps.

"We'd have to work awfully damn hard to deny these circumstances. Where does she think we'd get that kind of energy?"

"Beats me," I answered, hungry all of a sudden. Foregoing a knife and fork, I picked up my pork chop.

"What does she *do* while she's here? Does she see you taking care of Gus? Does she see you figuring out how to get rides to appointments when I can't get out of work?"

"Sometimes we take the buggy out and walk as we talk, and sometimes she walks us to the store so I can pick up a few things."

"Maybe she should do more of that and give up on the textbook stuff. I'm telling you Beth, these people have a solution in search of a problem." Mike was rolling to one of his boils. He took a quick drink of water and continued. "When I left this morning you were fine, Gus was happy, and you had the whole day in front of you. I come home and you look like hell. You don't need an MSW to see that what we need is help with the basics, like getting him to his appointments. If she can't see that, she's the one who's in denial, not us."

This wasn't anything I didn't already know. But between going blind and having Gus, my confidence was flagging. And we had always tended to believe the people who were supposed to help, like the Department of Rehabilitation Services counselor and the Braille Jail staff.

This time I demanded a different social worker. The replacement was great. She asked *me* what *I* thought I needed. Can you imagine? And eventually I asked the Public Health Department to quit sending out a nurse every week. These weren't easy requests, but they served as my first steps toward realizing that I knew more about our son, and about my own life, than any stranger could.

When Gus turned three, responsibility for special services shifted to the local public schools, as mandated by federal law. Gus actually began riding a bus (in his wheelchair) for half-days at school.

Other parents of disabled children had counseled us to be on guard—to demand what Gus had coming to him, not to let the

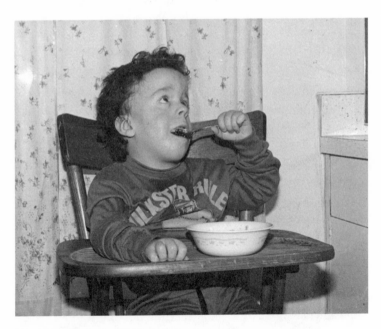

Five-year-old Gus in his high chair at home, 1991.

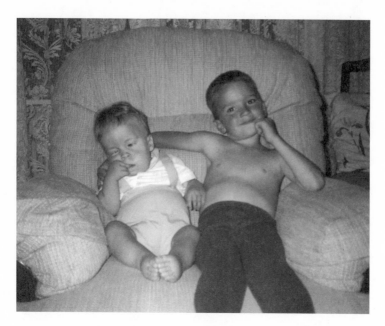

Gus hangs out with his cousin Robbie, 1988.

schools push us around. Well, I say, for all the flak teachers take, give 'em all a raise. We'd have been lost without the public schools; we probably would have had to institutionalize Gus at a very early age. Having him spend time outside our home freed me up to resume my rehabilitation and rebuild my life. And it gave Gus a chance to be a part of something beyond our little family unit. It has meant, too, that Mike and I haven't been alone in the struggles we face raising Gus.

———   ———

Not that there haven't been conflicts and disappointments. One of the stranger battles had to do with teaching Gus sign language. More than one speech therapist was hot on the idea, so eager to help Gus communicate that they forgot I couldn't see. Gus never did well with signing, and I wasn't willing to hold his hands twenty-four hours a day on the odd chance that he might formulate a word. There were so many other things the school could work on that *would* help us: toileting, grooming, and eating independently. I finally put my foot down, and we officially abandoned signing.

Another problem is that, in general, there never seems to be enough of the various therapists' time to go around. Vision specialists are in especially short supply. Gus can see well enough to find his cup on the kitchen table and to navigate our house in his wheelchair. He can spin that thing on a dime and roll around amazingly well. But I'm told he never looks at things straight on. He seems to look out of the corner of his eye. As he reaches for his cup, he's usually looking in another direction. When he was still small enough to sit on my lap, he liked to put his hand on my mouth when I sang to him. I would, in turn, search for his face and touch his mouth, hoping he might sing back to me. By feel I could tell that he was turned away, facing somewhere else. Yet he'd consistently zero in and grab my lower lip.

How he manages all this has always been a mystery to both medical doctors and therapists. Maybe because of my predicament, I'm especially eager for him to see as well as he possibly can. But between school budget limitations and shortages of trained personnel, visual specialists have been the missing link in all three school systems where Gus has been enrolled.

Apart from that general problem, our worst experience was in a district in a Chicago suburb. By 1994, Mike's job at Spyglass had evolved from technical writing to marketing communications. The company had grown, and when corporate headquarters relocated to Naperville, we moved.

We found a house in a nearby community and moved in November. Because Gus hadn't been a part of the local school's plan at the beginning of the year, he was bused forty-five minutes away to a school that had space for him. In the spring there was room for him locally, and things went well.

But in 1996, he started displaying behavioral problems. He'd throw hour-long fits, screaming, crying, banging his head and sometimes even biting himself and his caretakers. This was out of character. Not that he'd ever been a saint—he could throw a tantrum with the best of them when asked to do something that wasn't his idea. But he'd never been violent, and the tantrums had never lasted so long.

In the middle of all this, the school's physical therapist suggested Gus was ready for a new wheelchair. He had pretty much outgrown his old one, so we took the suggestion. The therapist took measurements and said she'd get the ball rolling. We gave her insurance information and waited for the next step. With no further consultation, the new chair arrived.

It was nice enough as wheelchairs go, but big and unwieldy. I struggled with it from the start. It didn't fit easily in the back of our station wagon as the old one had; Mike had to partly disassemble it each time we took Gus on an outing. And it was loaded with every feature imaginable, including multiple restraint devices.

A well-intentioned but overzealous therapist, we thought at first. Later we realized the chair was a response to Gus's behavior problems. Because it had restraints and could be tilted back recliner-style, Gus could be strapped in and parked until his tantrums subsided.

I understand the school's situation, but the episode still irks me. We ended up with a much more expensive chair than we needed. The bill was over five thousand dollars; our share, after insurance payments, was about twelve hundred. But even if insurance had covered the full amount, it shouldn't have had to. Worst of all, the chair wasn't a good solution to Gus's problem.

That solution didn't materialize for nearly a year. During a visit with Gus's old doctor in Urbana, we described his problems. The doctor thought Gus might be suffering from acid reflux. He prescribed a medication. Within a day the tantrums ended. Our lives improved immensely, but we had that damn chair until Gus finally outgrew it.

Babysitters were hard to come by during our years in the suburbs. Without a large university nearby, there was no pool of special education majors to draw on. Many suburban teens were too busy with extracurricular activities to have time to babysit; others were understandably leery of watching a ten-year-old in diapers. And most suburban kids simply didn't need the money. Our offers of high hourly pay (Mike's salary had increased significantly when we moved) were an insufficient lure.

We had made a point of finding a house in a town with a bank, a post office, many stores, and even a commuter rail line within walking distance. These features allowed me to stay fairly independent, and I made a point of getting out of the house regularly while Gus was at school. I knew Gus and I would be stuck at home from the time the school bus returned until Mike got home, most nights not until at least eight o'clock.

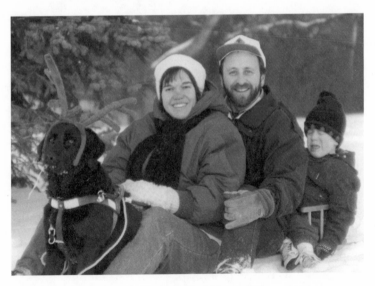

Holiday Greetings from Pandora, Beth, Mike, and Gus, ca. 1992.

Somehow Mike and I had managed to get wired into the 1990s version of the suburban American dream. Spyglass grew, and Mike hired a handful of people to work with him; he and his staff produced annual reports, maintained the Spyglass Web site, and coordinated appearances at the burgeoning Internet trade shows. Mike often flew to Boston, San Jose, or New York, leaving me with Gus. Flo and my sisters Bobbie and Cheryl lived forty minutes away and often checked in on us; Mike's boss's wife usually made it a point to stop by while Mike was away, too. In the mornings, however, I was on my own—waking, bathing, diapering, feeding, and dressing Gus, attaching his leg braces and lifting him into his wheelchair. I took special pride in having him ready each day when the school bus arrived.

Mike's long hours and hard work paid off. Spyglass became a mouse that roared during the Internet boom. Underfunded, understaffed, and against all odds, the company went public in June, 1995. Suddenly those pieces of paper that Mike had received in lieu of benefits and competitive salary became valuable. So valuable that Mike could quit working altogether for a while.

When Mike was deciding whether or not to leave Spyglass, we considered various options. If he stuck it out, perhaps we could save enough to put Gus in a private facility. A little research put an end to this idea; the private places—tranquil, leafy campuses where the rich and famous send their mentally retarded kids—cost $40,000 to $60,000 a year. Our good fortune had us looking at a lot of money according to our own standards, but not enough to put us in that league. We came to realize that Mike could continue working long hours, spending not much time with Gus and me, saving for a goal that would forever elude us.

That's when we chose the beach.

———

Mike quit his job, we sold our suburban house and took a temporary retirement in Nags Head, North Carolina. Every day Mike got to do something he'd dreamed of: take Gus to the bus each morning, and be there when it brought him back each afternoon. I got to share a leisurely morning coffee with Mike, sitting on the deck, listening to the waves and to Mike's hollers of joy when he spotted dolphins making their way past the Outer Banks.

The schools in our beach town had impressive new buildings and a reputation for strong parent involvement and energetic teachers. But when it came to special education, they were playing catch-up. Gus's teacher had not been trained in special ed. She had been passed over for a principal's position, we learned, and this new position wasn't her idea.

Still, Gus enjoyed some of his best school years ever at the beach. If his teacher had any problems with her position, she kept it to herself.

Cynthia Fields was African-American, a single mom of a teenage girl getting ready for college. What she lacked in special ed training was outweighed by her energy and her spirit. She was consistently upbeat, with a big voice that Gus responded to unlike any before or since. She laughed, she touched, she got on Gus for the bad and she praised him extravagantly when he learned something new. And she hugged him; we could smell her perfume on him on most days after school.

During his years in Cynthia Fields's class, Gus became more social, more curious, and more assertive. He learned to use a walker and he tooled around our beach house, laughing out loud every time he managed to find me or Mike and hug us. He liked going in the ocean, loved sitting on the deck, taking in the breeze and listening to the waves.

Maybe he was about to change anyway. Maybe it was because Mike and I spent more time with him, or that we were in high spirits. Or maybe he's a beach bum at heart. We'll never know. But in my book, it was Cynthia.

Our time on the beach was fabulous, full of simple pleasures.

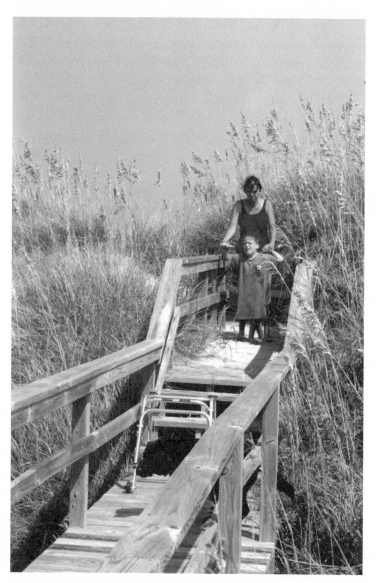

Gus and I approach the shore at Nags Head.

Without worrying about obstacles in my path, I was able to run by myself. Listening for the waves, I'd point my shoulders in their direction and spring toward them like a little girl. Sometimes Dora and I would race; she always won.

When the cold and rain arrived in December, Mike stoked the fireplace and I spent quiet time working on my writing. Mike took the occasional freelance consulting job, but mostly he puttered.

The dream ran its course. Before we left Illinois, I wanted to believe I was the type of woman who would be forever happy living by the ocean: listening to books, sitting by the fire, taking daily walks on the beach. Hard as it was to admit, I'm not that romantic figure. Two years of dreamy isolation were enough for me.

We made lovely friends on the Outer Banks, but we all lived far apart, and Nags Head had no public transportation. No sidewalks, either, which meant Dora and I were unable to do errands alone. Mike was responsible for grocery shopping, banking, mailing packages at the post office, taking us to appointments. He had the time, and mostly he seemed to enjoy it. But I started feeling dependent and disabled.

It's funny. On the beach or in the water, I enjoyed more of a sense of freedom of motion than at any other time since going blind. But the sound of the waves, the smell of the salt air, the feel of the sea on my skin . . . as fantastic and unforgettable as it all was, the ability to do all the other things by myself was more important.

We left the ocean in 1999 and moved back to Urbana. We now own the very house where, years ago, Mike and I sat on the porch swing and watched the sun go down.

———

Gus is now fifteen, weighs about a hundred pounds, and attends middle school. His teacher, Larry, is the lucky guy who's shared in Gus's exploits for the last couple years. Larry is a wonderful teacher, up to challenges. Gus has made great progress learning to use the toilet some during the last couple of years; you can't imagine the difference this makes to us. Larry has also managed to teach Gus to get in and out of his wheelchair. And he has worked with Mike on behavioral remedies for Gus's adolescent "explorations," the idea being to teach the notion that certain behaviors have appropriate times and places.

Each school-day morning I e-mail Larry about Gus's evening, how he slept, how much he ate and drank for breakfast. Larry usually writes me in the afternoon to sketch out Gus's day at school. All this communication helps with Gus's toilet program, and staying in sync helps us cope with behavior problems. We also get clues as to whether Gus might be getting sick. Because he can't talk, we often don't know he's caught a bug or come down with an ear infection

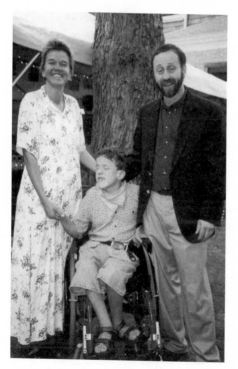

Our family at an outdoor celebration, 2000.

(which he's prone to, despite having ear tubes) until he's seriously ill. If he's consistently cranky, we can take him in to the doctor before things get too bad.

——— ———

When all four of us—Gus, Dora, Mike, and I—drive somewhere, it's quite the drill.

First there's Gus. We like to be sure that he's been on the toilet before we leave home, minimizing the chance of a nasty accident while we're away. Either Mike or I lift Gus onto the toilet seat, then stay in the room with him five to ten minutes. Gus doesn't much like sitting on the toilet; he'll immediately grab onto the sink next to him to pull himself up. Mike or I gently nudge him back where he belongs. When we get results (about one out of four times), Mike lifts Gus's arms into the air, crying out like Muhammad Ali, "You are the greatest!" I clap, sing, and do the dance of joy. Gus gets washed and has a new diaper put on; also a clean shirt if we're going out.

Around the house Gus often wears part of his last meal, particularly if I'm the one who fed him last. He wears a big kitchen dishtowel as a bib whenever I feed him, but it offers only so much protection. Before we leave, Mike checks Gus's clothing to see if it's fit for public viewing. We'll also check his bandana. Gus wears one under his chin because he drools so much.

While one of us finishes with Gus, the other goes to the back porch to retrieve Gus's collapsible transport chair (sort of a cross between a wheelchair and a stroller). Although his conventional wheelchair is better for his posture, the transport chair is lightweight; it rolls well over cracks and bumps; and it folds easily. After rolling the chair to the bathroom door, one of us—usually Mike—pulls Gus to standing, walks him to his chair, and with a grunt boosts his hundred pounds up and into the seat.

If it's not cold, I'm content to let Gus go out without shoes. Mike is not: "Gus should wear shoes, just like any other teenager." Since he's the one who feels strongly about this, he's usually the one to force shoes onto Gus's block-shaped feet. If it *is* cold, we put on Gus's coat and hat. He helps a little, raising his arms and poking his hands through his sleeves. One of us grabs his sippy cup (Gus can't drink from a normal cup without spilling) and a snack. He rarely needs the food, though; we always feed him before we go out so we can focus on enjoying our meal.

With Gus good to go, I take stock of myself, making sure I have my insulin pen. Mike checks for his keys and wallet, and at last we're ready to leave—unless Mike notices something amiss about my ensemble. (In the course of our preparations, I often ask Mike to confirm that I indeed am wearing what I think I'm wearing, and if so, that my clothes are clean. I have systems, but they're not failsafe.) I don't envy Mike at the times when he notices a spot on my shirt, my skirt inside out, or mismatched socks. My mistakes make me feel stupid and childish. More often than I like to think, I pout and lash out, shooting the messenger.

Mike escapes to the car, backing it down our driveway to the front entrance while I stomp back to my closet to straighten out my clothing.

Properly attired, I call Dora, leash her, and take her out to "empty," as The Seeing Eye puts it. Then her harness goes on and she leads me to the car. Meanwhile, Mike has been rolling Gus out the front door and onto the porch. (I used to push Gus onto the porch, but my technique of using the front wheels of the transport chair as feelers gashed our doorways and walls so badly that Mike has taken over this task.)

Mike rolls the chair down the ramp and to the rear door of our station wagon, then guides Gus—who can take steps awkwardly while leaning on Mike—into a position where his rear end faces the back seat. With a little push, Gus settles back next to Dora, who by now has nestled on the other side of the seat. Mike swings Gus's feet into the car and fastens his shoulder belt. Mike collapses the transport chair and hoists it into the cargo compartment.

"OK, we're here," Mike says once we've parked. He's been announcing our arrivals this way ever since the time I opened the car door at an intersection—we'd been at the red light so long that I assumed we'd reached our destination.

Sometimes handicapped parking is available, sometimes not. Mike gives me a mental map of our position. If it's on a one-way street, for example, and I'm on the traffic side, he'll tell me this and ask me to wait for him to come around before opening the door. In a parking lot, he warns me about when and how wide to open my door.

Once I'm safely out of the car, we both go to work on Gus, reversing the process we followed at home: Mike takes out the transport chair, unfolds it, and situates it near Gus's door. I remove Gus's seat belt, shift him so that his feet are near the pavement, then grab his hands and encourage him to stand. I reach out with my left hand to find the seat of his transport chair and place Gus's left arm around my neck, his hug giving me leverage. I say "Ready?" and then boost Gus into his chair with a loud grunt. (While appreciating my efforts, Mike often grows impatient watching our ritual and steps in to lift Gus himself.) With Gus settled in his transport chair, I call Dora to jump out of the back seat.

Then the parade begins. Mike pushes Gus's chair; Dora follows with me in tow. Years ago Mike joked that we must look like "Baby Elephant Walk." He still thinks it's funny to whistle that tune as we march down the street.

Mike enjoys dining at the same old restaurants. He knows they'll have easy access, big tables, wide aisles. Staff become accustomed to our drill and can function as his helpers. Hosts and hostesses know exactly where to seat us; servers ask questions of me, rather than directing them all to Mike; it's understood that Gus won't be eating, and it's no big deal.

Mike reads the menu aloud. (I try to anticipate what I might want so I can narrow him down to a certain category: just salads, maybe, or something with seafood. Otherwise it becomes awfully confusing, like hearing a recitation of the daily specials only more so.) My insulin kicks in after about thirty minutes. When we order, I quickly calculate how many units I'll need, based on my selection. I rotate a button on my insulin pen an appropriate number of clicks, unveil the needle, and discreetly shove it through my clothing and into my thigh.

We fill the sippy cup from our water glasses and set it where Gus can reach it. People stare at us more than I realize, I suppose; Mike rarely mentions this anymore. Gus loves restaurants, seems to enjoy the din of plates and silverware from the kitchen, likes to hear other patrons conversing. He claps, coos, and squeals with delight.

Staff who know us automatically tell me where things are when the food and drink is served. Mike locates salt, pepper, and other condiments if I need them. He alerts me when my water glass has been refilled or moved, and warns me when I mistakenly push food over the edge of my plate toward my lap. If a waiter has forgotten something, I have to ask Mike to flag him down.

We rarely visit a salad bar or brunch buffet. "Going to a restaurant is one thing, but buffet places make me feel like I'm an employee," he complains.

If I need to use the restroom, Dora can guide me if we're at a familiar place and I know where to point her. In an unfamiliar setting, other women on their way to the restroom are often happy to help guide us. If there are none, Mike scopes out the path and instructs me. When Dora and I make a wrong turn, he calls out a cue. In a pinch, he'll accompany us all the way there; I feel the eyes of our fellow patrons following us. When I open the door, he peeks in quickly and clues me in about where the toilets might be.

If I manage to find a toilet with the seat already down, I consider it a victory. Dora squeezes in the stall with me. On a day when everything is going right, a full roll of toilet paper awaits within arm's reach.

I skip the handwashing part. Locating sinks, soap dispensers, paper towels and garbage cans is all too much for me. Instead, I carry handwashing lotion.

Mike and I have been changing diapers for fifteen years now. We've also been feeding Gus, dressing him, walking him to the toilet, lifting him in and out of the car for outings and appointments. We're both plagued by back strain, but we manage. I take the occasional weekend to visit friends or family. Mike worries about leaving us overnight, but once in a while he takes his motorcycle out and spends the night in a state park, or catches a White Sox game and stays over in Chicago. When we manage overnights away from Gus—together or alone—we're reminded of what it's like to get a full night's sleep. Gus still often wakes two or three times a night, crying for a glass of water or words of comfort.

I am ready now to have Gus live outside our home in some sort of facility for the disabled, but Mike needs more time. To him, Gus is more lovable than ever. Gus has more personality and manages to express himself, at least to us and others who understand him. He makes it clear when he's hungry, and he can amble his awkward way to the kitchen table. When he wants to go outside, he gets to the door.

After the Spyglass boom, Mike bought himself an upright string bass and took lessons. I've switched from playing old-time music to jazz, and the two of us often jam together in the living room. Sometimes Gus joins in. Pulling himself onto the piano bench next to me, he fingers notes in time with us. He sings, too. Certain tones really catch his fancy, and he'll match them. He'll play a little back-and-forth game with me, matching a note I sing, or even singing along with me as my pitch rises and falls.

We're working with the school to take advantage of this skill, trying to get Gus to use it as a communication tool. His first tactic, when he wants something, is to whine. We typically have to wait him out, giving him attention only after he travels to the kitchen, or the screen door, or whatever he wants. Our hope is that he'll learn to sing out a pleasant tone when he wants help. So far it hasn't worked, but we're trying.

I got off to a rocky start with Gus. He wasn't what I imagined or wanted in a child, and he certainly made things more difficult and complicated for Mike and me. But we've come a long way. I love our little boy.

From the start, Mike adored Gus. Until recently, I think, he intended to keep Gus with us for as long as we live. At first this caused

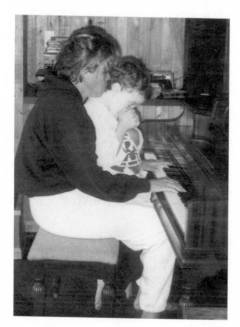

Gus and I enjoy making music together, 1998.

some friction between us. We had very different ideas about the future. But as Gus has grown and we have aged, Mike and I have gradually inched together. We both know we can't keep him forever.

We've already started investigating spots near Urbana, in and around Chicago, even in North Carolina. The day of the big institution is largely over—though that varies from state to state, and Illinois doesn't happen to shine in that regard. Still, more group homes have been established, and that's a good thing, though some house sixteen residents or more.

Kids like Gus simply aren't a high priority in our society. Professional staff members aren't paid particularly well; they burn out from all the paperwork, and from coping with extremely high turnover among the front-line staff, the ones who do the feeding and toileting and bathing, typically for the same wages paid to fast-food workers.

Still, we've met good people who do a remarkable job with minimal resources. Our priority is to find Gus a place near where we live, so we can visit frequently and unexpectedly. Other parents who've been through this tell us that staying involved is the single most important thing we can do. And we've learned—one bit of good news—that at least some kids seem happier once they leave home. I guess, in that way, they're like any other kids.

How I hope, when the time comes, it will turn out that way for our Gus.

8 | How I Do It

Gus isn't the only one who has changed and matured in the past fifteen years. My own life has evolved as well.

I had given up writing in 1980, after graduating from college, moving away from a career that had attracted me since childhood. (As a kid, I composed stories and compiled them into a newspaper that I sold door to door for a nickel. Newspaper publishing was fun, but the profits weren't good. *Neighborhood News* closed up shop after nine issues.) In 1971 I landed a writing position on the junior high newspaper; my beat was Homeroom 107. The high school paper was next, and at the University of Illinois I majored in journalism. Not until my final semester did I realize that I didn't want to be a journalist. Bothering people for interviews and stories was no fun.

I didn't start writing again until my eye surgeries failed. In the hospital I recorded my thoughts onto cassettes. Once home, I used an electric typewriter. My book project started at the end of 1987, when Mike presented me with a very special gift: a talking computer.

A handful of U.S. companies develop and market special screen-navigation software for blind people. Working in conjunction with a speech synthesizer, the navigation tools allow a blind user to move around a computer screen with keystrokes, and to hear characters and words read aloud.

My first experience with such a system came in January 1986, after I'd left Braille Jail. The University of Illinois Rehabilitation Center made talking computers available to dyslexic students and faculty members, as well as to the visually impaired. Luckily for me, Janet Floyd, the administrator I'd met when I still had some sight, believed that people not affiliated with the university should be allowed to use these machines whenever students and faculty members didn't need them. "It's your tax dollars," she reasoned.

I developed a routine: call Janet's office in the morning, find out when a computer would be available, then gather up my nerve to tap, tap, tap the eight blocks to the Rehab Center.

"We should get you a computer at home," Mike repeated daily.

"I think it's good that I have to walk. It forces me to use my cane."

Mike would sigh, cuss under his breath, then complain aloud that it was "goddamned insane." My eight-block journeys, which included one four-way stop, practically got him committed. I planned my getaways for times when he would be away from home and unable to offer a ride.

Fully aware of my stubbornness, Mike knew the only way he could pull off buying a computer would be to surprise me. At Christmas I was touched by all the trouble he'd gone through—the research, the money borrowed from Billy and Anne, the deliveries to neighbors so I wouldn't be suspicious—but miffed that he'd gone ahead without my approval.

There wasn't time to stay angry. With a computer at home, my hours were quickly consumed with transferring addresses and phone numbers from cassette to computer file, setting up a check register and a calendar I could access from the keyboard. Soon after that, my days started resembling those of my friends: seated in front of the keyboard, I made phone calls, wrote letters, scheduled appointments, worked on our budget. All of this without messing with Braille, fumbling with cassettes, or relying on Mike to read anything aloud.

I've had five different talking computer setups since then: a DOS machine, then a Mac, and since then a succession of Windows-based machines. I had to leave my keyboard for a moment just now to ask Mike the exact name of the computer I currently use: a Gateway machine with Windows 98 and a Celeron Processor. What all that means, I'm not sure; I just know it works. Mike's the one who stays abreast of the technologies, reads the manuals, makes sure I get the updates, and provides tech support.

The computer I used while writing this book works with a pocket-sized speech synthesizer that plugs into and out of any standard computer. The synthesizer calls out letters as I type so I can hear and fix my typos as I go. I manipulate keys to make it read a page of type by word, line, or paragraph when I want to check spelling and grammar. Although advances in technology have improved the quality of the synthesized voice, friends insist it still sounds like something out of a science fiction movie and wonder aloud how I "can understand that thing."

In 1999 an essay of mine appeared in our local alternative weekly. After that I was asked to contribute regularly. This boosted my confidence and motivated me to write freelance pieces for other magazines.

When it comes to reporting, the "411" information number helps me to locate phone numbers so I can arrange interviews. (Because telephone books aren't much good to the blind, the phone company lets us use 411 free of charge.) Mike drives me to do story interviews when he can. At other times I take cabs or buses, or walk with Dora.

I use a talking keyboard as my date book—it's screenless, which makes it small and easy to carry. My talking watch and the hourly church chimes in town keep me on time for appointments.

Like many other reporters, I tape interviews with a standard handheld tape recorder. I tape phone interviews (always forewarning subjects, of course) using a little microphone from Radio Shack. With a slate-and-stylus device I punch Braille dots onto labels, then attach them to the cassettes.

Mike reads finished stories aloud to me before I send them off. It's easier to catch syntax errors listening to his human voice than to the robotic drone of my talking computer—plus he usually catches a few errors. I use my talking computer to e-mail finished pieces to publishers. Editors review the stories and reply via e-mail with corrections.

Of course, I'm always excited when a magazine or newspaper accepts one of my pieces. Then sadness mixes with my joy when it is published and I can't see it in print. (I tell myself this must be how Beethoven felt after losing his hearing.) Mike reads my published works aloud to me, doing his best to describe the page layout and accompanying artwork. With the help of a scanner, I can transfer these works to my computer and have the speech synthesizer repeat them to me later. When stories appear on-line, my computer can read those, of course. I'm grateful to Mike (to anyone I can recruit as a reader, for that matter), and I realize that I'm privileged to have access to technology for the blind. Truth is, though, it just ain't the same as reading a printed page. In fact, one of the things I miss most from my seeing days is scanning a newspaper. Whenever I go out for coffee, I find myself envying the folks around me, rustling a paper in one hand, clinking their cappuccino cup against its saucer with the other.

I'm lucky to live in an age when so much material is available on tape or compact disc. Proud, too, to be living in a country where the Library of Congress has for seventy years offered recorded books to the blind, free of charge. Most of my books on tape come from the National Library Service for the Blind and Physically Handicapped. I was first given one of their special tape players during a hospitalization for eye surgery. Since then, I've received recorded books simply by calling an 800 number and ordering them. The NLS tapes come in special containers; when I've finished listening, I simply flip over an address card and drop the whole thing into any mailbox, gratis. Because I can listen to books while I do laundry, wash dishes, feed Gus and all that, I read more books now than when I could see.

The National Library Service records the same sorts of books that public libraries carry in print. As happens with a regular library, often the books I request are unavailable. In some cases they've been checked out; in others, they've simply never been recorded. Over the years, generous friends have taken time to record some relatively obscure books for me. A friend from my diabetic support group records every new diabetic memoir that comes out—many of these would never gain the popularity necessary for the Library of Congress to bother with them. My friend Brad regularly reads and records sections of *Writer's Market* so I'll know which magazines accept freelance articles. Volunteers read aloud from the three-ringed notebook of reference materials I received when training for a hospice group.

Many of these same people, along with students from two service organizations at the university, sort through and read aloud the pile of mail, newsletters, and newspaper articles that I accumulate each week. Recently a friend began to home school her twelve-year-old. "Could one of his assignments involve reading to a blind person?" I asked. "Of course," she said. He comes once a week, reads the paper aloud, and we discuss current events.

When I became serious about publishing the book you're now reading, I paid Audio Studios for the Reading Impaired to have one person read my text aloud into a microphone while another listened for mistakes. This organization, based in Kentucky, required two copies of my manuscript and a small fee based on the number of pages read and the number of cassettes used.

As for reading Braille, my skills remain at a first-grade level; it takes about a half-hour for me to make sense out of a page of Braille dots. I use Braille to label things like CDs and spice jars, but that's about it. The NLS provides books in Braille form, but I've never ordered one. It'd be nice to read fast enough to interpret books in my own voice again rather than relying on a reader; tempting though this prospect may be, I've never mustered the energy to take any more Braille courses. It's just too easy to listen to books on tape.

After losing my sight I missed writing and receiving letters. E-mail changed all that. With the help of my talking computer and a set of headphones, I can transmit and listen to e-mail whenever I feel like it. Even if I'm interrupted midstream, I can return to the note later; this had been impossible back when I used an electric typewriter, for I had no way to read anything I'd just written and never knew where I'd left off.

E-mail also relieves me of the cumbersome task of addressing envelopes. I still own a special clipboard with a movable straight edge to help me print legible addresses, but I rarely use it now.

Before e-mail, cassette tapes served as my only means for corresponding without a sighted reader. Lots of my friends never grew comfortable speaking on tape, but for the few who did, the habit has stuck. Mike and I often tape messages to these friends together, especially in the car during long trips. The U.S. Postal Service allows the visually impaired to send cassettes, Braille, or large-print materials postage-free. Of course, snail mail also works for gifts and other packages. I love packing them myself. Then I print the address from a computer file onto a sheet of paper and take it along to the post office. Postal workers who have struggled to make out my handwriting are more than happy to label my boxes for me.

I like keeping up with old friends, and I used to enjoy throwing big parties to gather them in one place. With six older brothers and sisters, just sitting down for dinner every night seemed like a party when I was a kid. We regularly had shindigs in our basement, and every Fourth of July my trombonist brother, Doug, got his jazz friends together for an outdoor blast in our backyard, shoving the piano out from our living room onto the driveway for the event. Flo spooned out sloppy joes onto hamburger buns, and I ceremoniously presented these mountains of sandwiches to the crowds. While I was in high school and college there were annual polka parties in our yard, and Flo never missed a dance. Everyone knew that if you threw a big party, those Finkes would be there.

Truth be told, big parties aren't much fun for me now. Small get-togethers—six people or fewer—are the way to go; with more than that, I find it too tricky and exhausting to follow multiple conversations.

Even with Dora at my side, I'm at something of a disadvantage when it comes to schmoozing. In an unfamiliar environment, I can't direct her, so someone has to guide us. Mike is patient about playing that role, and so are friends, but sticking with one person can defeat the major purpose of a party, which is to mingle.

Early on in my blindness, another guest cornered me at a party. She wasn't a bad person, just didn't know when to quit talking. In my seeing days, I'd have escaped by going for food, or saying I wanted to freshen my drink, or whatever. I tried excusing myself to head to the bathroom, but she insisted on guiding me, talking all the way, then waiting and chauffeuring me back to our original spot. Her chatter started acting like a vise on my head—it's what I imagine claustrophobia to be like.

Finally, I exploded. I pointed my face toward the ceiling and shouted Mike's name into the air. Worried, he came running and rushed me outside, where he was relieved to hear I wasn't ill, just feeling trapped. Nowadays at parties Mike checks on me periodically.

"You OK?" he'll ask. If I need a break, I'll answer by grabbing his elbow, so he knows to guide me away and park me in a new spot. Other hand signals now substitute for our old visual cues. A shift of Mike's eyes toward the exit used to indicate boredom; now his firm grasp on my knee under a table lets me know he's ready to leave. Mike has learned to poke me sharply three times to let me know that the very person I'm gossiping about is standing right next to me. If I'm not within striking distance, he calls out "Poke, poke, poke!" from across the room.

Instead of visiting with friends at parties, I like to take long walks with them. I'm especially happy when the walk ends up at a coffee shop or a tavern.

———

In fact, it's not unusual for me to travel quite a great distance to visit an old friend. Since Gus was born, I've flown to the Yucatan Peninsula and to Belfast, and I've used trains and buses to travel across the United States.

Air travel with Dora is surprisingly easy. Our first flight out of Newark was also Dora's and my very first solo venture after graduating from The Seeing Eye. Miss Early accompanied us through the terminal to the gate, talking me through the security check routine while we waited in line. "I'll put your bags on the conveyor belt," she said. "Then Pandora will lead you to the detector. Have her sit there, then let go of her harness and walk through, holding only the leash." Then I was to command Pandora to come. "She'll beep because of her harness. They may have to use the wand to check her, but it'll save them doing that to you, too." This procedure worked beautifully that day, perhaps because the security guards were used to guide dogs.

In public situations, things consistently go more smoothly if people think I'm alone with Dora. Otherwise the airline people talk to my human partner, rather than addressing me directly—they look to the "normal" traveler to take care of everything. If we're at the security check, confusion can ensue. Dora and I may be led far from the detector to have the wand run over us. Travelers behind us grow impatient as my companion attempts to marshal our bags as they come off the rollers.

When Dora and I travel alone, or when (as Mike and I have started doing lately, for the sake of convenience) my companion and I pretend not to be together, people are forced to deal with me. I always manage; they always manage; Mike is freed from being responsible for me and my belongings. It's downright liberating, all the way around.

Dora has flown with me so often that she can guide me down the jetway and into the plane by herself. We follow a flight attendant to our seat, which is often at the bulkhead, sparing Dora the cramped conditions beneath a seat in front of us. Dora is always remarkably calm on planes.

Train travel goes roughly the same way. Dora guides me up the steps to the train car, but without flight attendants to greet us we're left to find an empty seat on our own. "Is this spot free?" I ask when Dora turns to a seat. If no one answers, I know we're safe to sit.

Once we reach our destination, Dora guides me from the train to the station. It always scares me a bit. Trains are loud, and it's difficult to hear if we're heading in the right direction. Accounts of blind people falling onto subway tracks don't ease my state of mind. Even with the bumpy warning surfaces that have been installed at platform edges in most stations, I'm fearful. I try to limit train travel to Amtrak and commuter lines; when I must take subways, I try to enlist a sighted guide to accompany Dora and me.

When it's too far to walk, cabs are a convenient alternative. (Although once or twice drivers have balked at accommodating Dora.) You can't beat door-to-door service, but it doesn't come cheap, so mostly I stick with buses. My early attempts, back when I was using a cane, weren't terribly successful. On my first try, after I'd found my way to a corner and waited patiently, the bus drove right past me. Because I hadn't been looking toward it as it approached, the driver must have thought I was simply waiting to cross the street. Now I stand only at marked stops and always face the approaching bus. Before I get on I ask the driver to confirm the number or route. Then I enlist the driver as my helper, saying where I'd like to get off, and Dora leads me to an open seat. Most drivers call out significant intersections so I can track our progress.

My favorite way to get around town is on foot. Dora's fun to walk with, I enjoy the exercise, and I'm too impatient to waste time at bus stops if I can avoid it. Besides, Seeing Eye dogs should walk three miles every day to keep in good shape.

Taking care of Dora is by no means easy, but it's not a burden when I consider all she does for me. She eats high-grade dry dog food, which Mike buys in big bags from a local feed store. (The students from my Seeing Eye class who live alone with their guide dogs tell me they have volunteers pick up food for them or have it delivered by UPS or U.S. Mail.) I use a plastic cup to measure out Dora's food twice a day; she also receives a daily dose of buffered aspirin for minor arthritis pain. I pry her mouth open with one hand and place the pill on the back of her tongue with the other—quite an accomplishment for someone who used to be afraid of dogs. I also pry her mouth open to brush her teeth, and I flip up her ears to wash them out with hydrogen peroxide and water now and then.

Dora goes through an obedience ritual every day to remind her of basic commands: "Rest," "Heel," "Come," and "Fetch."

I heft Dora's water bowl from the floor throughout the day to feel that it's full. At least four times a day I call her to the back door, attach her leash, and take her out to empty. Even Seeing Eye dog owners who have fenced yards take their dogs out on leashes. Without seeing the dogs, we can't know whether they're sneaking out over or under a fence, nor can we see what flora or fauna they might covet.

Being attached by leash also alerts us when the dog is pooping. Dora walks around in countless circles before finding exactly the right spot. When she finally stops circling, I feel for her back. If it's rounded, I know she's squatting. Placing my foot near her tail, I slip a plastic bag over my right hand and reach down. I feel the ground through the bag until I encounter some lumps, pick them up, fold the bag over my palm, and that's that. We were taught this technique at The Seeing Eye, for all the obvious reasons. I hate stepping in dog shit and complain profanely any time I do. I wouldn't feel right complaining about the negligence of other dog owners if I didn't pick up after Dora. Besides, picking up after her consistently is a good way to make sure she isn't sick or hasn't eaten anything rotten.

I brush Dora's coat each day so she doesn't shed in public or at friends' homes. Grooming gives me a chance to check her for lumps or other irregularities. Twice a year I take her for a checkup. The Seeing Eye pays vet bills during the first year the dog is home; graduates are responsible for any medical expenses their dogs incur thereafter.

Anyone with a companion animal knows it's hard to predict how much a visit to the vet may cost. If I don't have enough cash along to pay Dora's bill, I either pull out a credit card or write a check. To sign the credit card slip in a straight line, I have the receptionist position something with a straight edge (a sturdy envelope, a checkbook cover) where I'm meant to sign. Given a pen, I scribble a signature. A special plastic template with window cutouts helps me stay in line when writing checks.

When it comes to cashing checks, the drill is similar to the one used with credit cards. My bank teller turns the check upside down and positions a straight-edge where I'm meant to sign. The teller hands me a pen; I scribble a signature.

I keep track of money by folding each denomination differently. I developed the following system: twenties are folded in half, tens down to three-quarter size. Fives get the end folded into a triangle and singles I just leave be. The teller calls out each bill as it's placed in my hand, then waits for me to fold it and put it in my wallet before presenting the next. I simply trust these tellers not to cheat me, and they don't let me down. I balance my own checkbook on my talking computer. It has a calculator function, but I add and subtract the old-fashioned way, in my head.

Mike and I have gone through plenty of money since I lost my sight. Besides the obvious medical bills, we've moved six times. We've frustrated a lot of real estate agents along the way.

"We have the perfect house for you," they'll say. "It's all on one floor, wide doorways for Gus's wheelchair, near town, even has a fenced-in yard for Dora!"

Then Mike and I arrive and realize there are no sidewalks. Or all the nearby stores are surrounded by parking lots that Dora and I can't negotiate safely. Or there are no stoplights to get us across a busy street.

We persevere, though. Aside from our move to North Carolina, I've always been able to do most of our shopping errands, leaving Mike responsible only for weekly groceries or the bigger purchases that require a car.

Before using Dora to guide me to stores in a new town, I enlist a sighted volunteer to walk me to shops I think I'll be frequenting, getting a feel for their locations. Otherwise I phone ahead and get directions. I need to know the approximate location of the store so I can tell Dora how to get there, when to go left, right, or forward. Corner stores are the easiest to find. To locate others, I quietly repeat "Right, right, right" or "Left, left, left" and motion toward where I think the door might be. The worst that can happen is Dora takes us into the wrong shop. I can usually tell if the doorknob feels unfamiliar or the smells and sounds inside aren't right.

Once in the right store, Dora takes me directly to the counter. If the clerk doesn't know us, I'm usually greeted with a "May I help you?" I've piped up so many times when this question was actually being asked of another customer that I've learned to point at myself and ask, "Us?" before answering. If the clerk happens to be in the back room or looking the other way, there's always the chance they're unaware of Dora at my feet. The "Us?" question really throws them. Then, when I ask for something right in front of my eyes, the clerk can really get annoyed. (I know by the tone of voice or the prolonged silence.) When they point somewhere and say, "It's right here!" I reply with my own pointing. "I can't see it," I say, directing my finger down toward Dora and her Seeing Eye harness. A flurry of apologies results.

It's worse when I leave Dora at home and walk into a store with a friend. Sometimes I get through a whole round of questions without a clerk realizing I'm blind; only when they hold out my change and I don't grab it do they discover something's fishy. I've learned to make a preemptive strike by holding my palm upturned to make the cashier place the money in my hand.

My favorite way to practice folding bills is by shopping for new clothes. Some people suppose that, if they lose their sight, they could finally forget about how they look. In fact, I am more concerned with my appearance now than I ever was as a sighted person. People watch me a lot now. Some are merely rude, but most are trying to be kind, looking out for me. They comment as I negotiate steps, call out directions when I lean down from my bus seat to fetch my backpack. I can't help suspecting that they also notice my appearance. If my clothes don't match or if something isn't tucked in properly, I imagine them thinking, *Poor thing, she doesn't realize.*

I don't like being pitied, so gone are those college days when I threw on whatever was in my closet and ran out the door. So are the days of rummaging through bins at discount stores and resale shops. Irony of ironies, now that I can't even see how I look, I shop at one of the pricier stores in town.

The first time I went there, I tried on a pair of tight leggings. "Honey," the owner said, "you've got some hips." She was right. I didn't buy the leggings, but I did become a faithful customer. The owner is honest about how things fit, whether they hang correctly, whether the colors are good. She even sets aside outfits that she thinks will flatter me. I don't own a lot of clothes now, but what I do have is made well and is easy to mix and match. If people are going to stare at me, I'd like them to be pleasantly surprised.

I pay attention to my hair for that same reason. At first I wanted it all cut off. "I don't want to deal with curling irons or electric rollers anymore," I told my hairdresser.

"Well, do you want to deal with makeup, then?" she asked. "Because if you don't have hair and you don't wear makeup, you're going to look like a boy."

Funny, I thought if I got my hair cut off I'd look like Annie Lennox.

My hairdresser and I came up with a compromise. I wear my hair short, in a cut where all I have to do is throw my head upside down, brush it from underneath, and let it fall back when I toss my head up again. And I wear no makeup—I just wash my face in the morning and hope for the best. So far, no one's complained.

Body hair is another story. Unsolicited comments about my unshaven armpits and legs finally shamed me into action. Home alone one day, I changed the blade on a razor myself and went to work, giving Mike the scare of his life when he returned: blood on the doorknobs, blood on the stereo, blood on the refrigerator. Unknowingly, I'd nicked my finger, and everything I'd touched after that was crimson.

Ever since that Lizzie Borden episode, I've used disposable razors.

I'm not sure what I look like anymore. I was a slim and trim twenty-six-year-old when I lost my sight. If I shower quickly, not pinching any inches along the way, I have the luxury of picturing myself that way even now. On the many days when I can't completely convince myself of this fantasy, I imagine that my well-chosen attire does wonders to hide any middle-aged spread.

The jig was up soon after I turned forty and my clothes started feeling tight. Apart from vanity, of course, weight is an important health issue—all the more so for diabetics. Grudgingly, I've learned to weigh myself. I shove the big weight on our old-fashioned scale to the right until it slips into the third groove: 150 pounds. If the balancing lever clunks downward on the right when I step on the scale, I'm golden. If it tips up, there's trouble.

After too many upward tips this year, I added more laps to my weekly regimen. Swimming back and forth in a pool is the easiest form of exercise for me. (Although it's hard on Dora. She whines, cries and pulls on the leash if I hook her up to the ladder at the edge while I swim. Hardly relaxing, for me or for other swimmers—not to mention for Dora, who wants both to swim and to save me from drowning. So I travel to the pool the old-fashioned way, tapping my white cane.)

The locker room is no trouble to negotiate: Nice smooth floors, easy to tap with my cane (because devoid of the cracks and other irregularities that catch the tip); aisles; shower stalls at predictable right angles. The towel ladies have assigned me an easy-to-find locker on the end of a row and kindly replaced the combination lock with one that uses a key. I undress, feel my swimsuit to make sure it's right side out, then squeeze it on. I assume the shower room walls have the usual signs: "All swimmers must take nude showers." I use blindness as an excuse to ignore them.

Though I already knew how to swim, just after I lost my sight I signed up for a "Swimming for the Handicapped" class at the university. I figured I might get some pointers about swimming straight without being able to see. My teacher, a graduate student in rehab therapy, taught the class in order to receive his tuition waiver.

The first day he offered his elbow and led me to the Olympic-sized pool. We were a small group, only four or five students; each of us received some one-on-one attention. Without being able to see the other students, I wasn't sure what their disabilities were. I could hear that one student was in a wheelchair and had to use a special lift to get in and out of the pool. Aside from that, I knew only that each of us got a private lane. At the university's popular intramural building, getting your own lane at the indoor pool was otherwise inconceivable.

I loved it, and I took advantage of it. My teacher stood behind me at the edge of the pool, grabbed my arms and pulled them up in the air. "Reach up as far as you can, then pull back toward your belly button. And concentrate!" I pushed off the side, concentrated, and banged right into a lane marker. I tried again, pushed off the side, and careened from one marker to the next, all the way down and back. I was an underwater missile with no guidance system. I needed that lane all to myself.

I never did learn to swim straight. I asked my teacher if I could tap each lane marker with my hand, just to keep my bearings. "It'll slow your pace," he warned—as though I actually cared about being competitive.

One evening, after a particularly hard workout, I pulled myself out of the pool, only to find him awkwardly silent. He usually offered enthusiastic coaching advice.

Finally he spoke. "You need to fix your suit," he said quietly. So quietly that I had to ask him to repeat it.

"You need to fix your suit," a little louder this time. I felt the seams and realized that my right boob had found its way into the open air. I shoved it back inside the fabric, grabbed my teacher's trembling elbow, and held on for dear life. He couldn't guide me over those wet tiles and to the women's locker room fast enough.

I received an "A" in the class. I swim three times a week now, tapping the lane marker with my right hand on every other stroke.

Between walking, swimming, and an occasional ride on the back of our tandem bicycle, I thought I was doing pretty well in terms of exercise. Then my longtime friend Mim Nelson, whom I'd met years earlier when I studied overseas, told me about a book she'd researched and written. Tremendously proud of Mim, I bought dozens of copies of *Strong Women Stay Young* and started giving the book to sisters, friends, and neighbors for birthdays and other special occasions.

As long as her book was only available on paper, I figured I had an excuse not to follow Mim's teachings. When the Library of Congress offered it on tape, the jig was up. Now, after listening to *Strong Women Stay Young,* I find myself a most unlikely weight lifter. Following Mim's taped directions, I work with free weights in the comfort of my own living room, often while listening to Terry Gross's "Fresh Air" interviews on National Public Radio.

———

It is my goal to be interviewed on radio or even TV, and I am eager to look my interviewer straight in the eyes when I answer each question. Teachers at Braille Jail taught us how to do this: "Figure out exactly where the voice is coming from, then look three or four inches up from there. If you look at people's eyes, they'll be more comfortable talking to you."

Mike was my coach. I practiced and practiced. Soon I could look him right in the eyes every time he spoke. When I tried this elsewhere, though, it didn't work. Others still seemed uncomfortable talking to me.

It was my right eye. It had shrunk after surgery, and I could barely hold my eyelid open. Mike had seen me like this for so long that he no longer noticed. As I mentioned earlier, I wasn't aware of how bad it looked until my niece Caren alerted me.

Where do you find a good glass-eye maker? I wondered.

Fortunately, the mother of a high school friend was an optometrist whose Chicago office shared a floor with an ocularist. "We don't call them glass eyes anymore," the ocularist told me on my first visit. "And they're never shaped like round marbles, the way people imagine." In cases like mine, he explained, where the eye globe is still intact (albeit small), a scleral shell prosthesis is constructed. Mine fits entirely over my own globe.

"It'll look like a natural eye," he said, "and it will hold your eyelid open."

All the time?

"No, you'll be able to blink as you normally would."

Normal is what I wanted.

First, my eye socket was filled with a goop called alganate. After forty-five seconds the alganate stiffened, forming an impression of my shrunken eye and the surrounding tissue. From that impression a two-piece mold was cast in dental stone. Molten wax was poured into the mold. When the wax hardened, it became the master for what was eventually my prosthesis. For two or three hours, the wax master was repeatedly inserted into my eye, taken out and tailored a bit. Meticulous effort is required to provide the proper direction of gaze, vertical and horizontal movement, and eyelid opening. The finished wax master was then put into a new mold of white acrylic.

Two weeks later I had a sitting with June, a professional artist who painted the acrylic mold to match my left eye. We chatted as she worked. I learned she had a graduate degree in painting but found it hard to pay the bills selling her artwork alone; painting eyes gave her a regular paycheck. "Doesn't allow for much creativity," she conceded. "But it does help me practice technique."

After three hours or so, June had seen me enough to finish without me. I made another appointment for my final fitting. At the third appointment June gave me a lecture on proper care for my prosthesis. I could leave it in all the time or take it out at night. If I took it out, I should store it in tap water and clean it with regular hand soap and water. Every once in a while I would need to come back and have it checked and polished.

She finally placed the eye in my hand.

"Try not to touch it too much," she warned. "The oils from your skin aren't good for the finish."

She directed my fingertip to a teeny-tiny hole toward the edge of the shell. "We put that hole there so you'll know which side goes down."

She asked me to lean forward. Holding my chin to steady my face, she used her free hand to spread the lids of my poor shrunken eye, then plopped the prosthesis in.

"OK!" she exclaimed. "It's in. It looks great."

Intellectually I knew the prosthesis wasn't meant to improve my eyesight; it would only enhance my looks. Subconsciously, though, I must've thought it would restore my sight. And here I was, still a blind woman. But at least a normal-looking blind woman. Now, when I wear the prosthesis and look at people when I talk, I often receive the confusing compliment that I "don't look blind."

———   ———

I didn't become a fabulous pianist the minute my eyesight vanished, and I don't spend every moment surrounded by music now, either. In fact, I rarely listen to the stereo. If I'm listening to the radio, I usually choose news or talk. Without being able to read the newspaper, radio offers the best way for me to keep up with what's happening. Were I to have music blasting on the stereo, I couldn't hear other, more important, noises. Like Gus clapping his hands, letting me know where he is. Or paper crinkling, telling me Dora's getting into food in the kitchen.

When I want to listen to music, I prefer hearing it live. I especially like small informal places; I can sit back with a cup of coffee or a beer, make comments to friends about what we're hearing without being scolded by those around us.

I no longer attend big concerts. They're too expensive, too loud. And really, half the fun at big rock concerts comes from people-watching, a form of entertainment I can no longer enjoy. Formal concerts, too, are unrewarding. Seated in a cushy seat at a concert hall, I don't seem to be able to feel the music the way I can in a smaller setting.

Lucky for me, an Urbana joint was recently converted to a small music club featuring local musicians and the occasional out-of-towner en route to a Chicago gig. The spot is within walking distance; some evenings we push Gus along in his wheelchair. Like me, Gus appreciates the difference between recorded music and the real thing. An enthusiastic fan, he claps, squeals, and shakes with excitement, nearly jumping out of his seat with joy at what he hears.

It doesn't hurt that this place serves free popcorn, too. Popcorn is one of my favorite foods. As I've mentioned, I must take insulin whenever I have something to eat. This might keep some people from eating very often. Not me—I like food too much. So every time the waitress places a basket of popcorn on our table, I grab my insulin and inject a couple of units into my thigh, right through my skirt or jeans.

Taking multiple shots a day became much easier for me in 1997, when I started using an insulin pen, rather than messing with syringes and vials. Any time I need a dose, I simply rotate the pen top, dial an appropriate number of clicks, and take a shot.

Eating proper meals without seeing presents few problems, although knives can be a little treacherous. I usually ask others to cut meat for me, rather than struggling with it myself. I let people cook for me, too—even sighted, I was a liability in the kitchen. Of course, because I do get hungry at times when I'm home alone, I make sure identifiable snacks are always on hand.

I actually do make bread from scratch. I learned how after helping with a local charity's phone-athon; at the end of the evening, we were offered the leftover snacks. "There's even a whole loaf of bread here," someone said.

At home, after removing the foil, Mike gave me the bad news: banana bread, too sweet for me to eat. "Take it to work tomorrow," I suggested. "Tell them your wife made it."

Ah, what a tangled web we weave. The bread was such a hit that Mike's co-workers wanted me to teach them how to make it. Matters only worsened when I called the phone-athon folks and discovered that the baker was, in fact, the church pastor. Determined to maintain my newfound image as Suzy Homemaker, I phoned the pastor and confessed my sin. He laughingly assured me that he'd come over and give me a baking lesson.

I've been baking bread ever since. The dough forming as I knead, the smell of the yeast as the loaf rises, the warmth of the oven on a cold day, the aroma of baking—these sensual experiences do not require vision. I control how much sugar is used, making it easier to determine how much insulin I'll need once I've thumped the bread to find out that it's ready.

Mike makes the weekly shopping runs. I'm in charge of stowing the groceries in the cupboards—that way I know where everything is. As I go, I ask Mike for help with any object I can't identify. I'll dent or stretch rubber bands around cans to differentiate them. Mike is consistent about the types of containers he buys: soda in cans, beer in bottles, juice in square cardboard containers, and milk in jugs.

Ordinarily I manage pretty well in the kitchen. To make oatmeal for Gus, for example, I scoop out dry oatmeal, hold the full cup above the oatmeal container, level it off with a knife, then dump the cup's contents into a cereal bowl. I run water into a one-cup measure until it starts to overflow, pour it in with the oatmeal, mix it a bit, set it in the microwave, and press the appropriate buttons, which are marked in Braille.

Routine and consistency are the keys. It's when outside influences intrude that havoc ensues. Take my first morning home with Pandora. Because I had failed to level off the dry oatmeal, it overflowed in the microwave. I shifted around while wiping it up, with Pandora's leash wrapped around my ankle, per Seeing Eye instructions for our first weeks together. I succeeded with the oatmeal preparations on my second try. Pandora guided me to Gus. I carried him to his highchair and wrapped Pandora's leash around my ankle again. I needed both hands to feed Gus. (Actually I needed about four hands.) Pandora kept slinking under Gus's highchair to clean up what he'd dropped, and she had to be corrected.

And so on. When it was finally my turn to eat, I punched the button on my talking clock. It was already ten thirty. I hadn't even had my coffee yet. I found coffee filters, ground the beans, and proceeded to make the worst pot of coffee I'd ever tasted. When Mike came home at noon, I was still in my pajamas. He didn't comment on that. He did, however, ask me why pinto beans were in the coffee grinder.

———

As if life weren't complicated enough with a dog and a baby at home, I also provided daycare of infants for a while to earn pocket money. I still care for my nieces' and nephews' babies from time to time.

Because infants don't move much, they're easy to keep track of. To pick them up, I place my hands palms down on the mattress and feel around until I find a little body, then figure out which end is which and lift the baby to my shoulder, one hand always under its head for support. I walk backward from room to room—that way if we bump into doorframes or walls, it's my well-padded bottom or my shoulders that bear the impact.

Most parents supply prepared bottles, which I can heat in the microwave. And yes, I always shake the bottle to make sure the formula isn't too hot.

When bathing a baby, I always have soap, shampoo, and towels within arm's reach so I can keep one hand on the baby while searching with the other. If a baby wants to stretch out, I lay it on a blanket on the floor. I never, ever step on this blanket, whether a baby is on it or not. This way I can keep small toys out all the time and not worry about tripping over them or stepping on the baby.

I learned all this taking care of Gus, of course. But now he crawls, even struts around our house using a walker. He loves percussion instruments, and I'm constantly kicking or stepping on the tambourines and drumsticks he leaves in his wake. He's taken to tapping on floors and walls as he moves about, so I always have a good idea where he is.

Gus crawls to the kitchen table, pulls himself up and taps on it when he's hungry or thirsty. He can drink from a sippy cup and eat finger food by himself. If we fill a fork or spoon with food, he can guide it to his mouth. Every little bit helps.

Still, anytime I'm helping Gus with food, it seems as much ends up *on* him as *in* him. I do a lot of laundry. We have layers of tape on our washer dials to mark temperatures and water levels; I memorize the dryer settings. Mike rubs stain remover on anything he catches that needs it. I wash everything in cold water so undetected stains are less likely to set. And with cold water I don't have to separate white things from colored.

Mike chooses to do his own laundry. He used to do most of the house cleaning, too, but never by choice. I would clean during the day and inevitably miss huge patches of grime or unknowingly shove hair balls into corners. Mike had the unhappy task of informing me of my failures. He hated seeing my reaction (I sometimes cried, I was so disappointed) and began quietly cleaning up after me instead. Eventually he started resenting all the work. Fights ensued. We finally looked hard at our budget and found a way to hire house cleaners.

Like the students who volunteer to read to me and take me on errands, the folks who have cleaned for us over the years have become our friends. Right now we employ a Brazilian couple, here to learn English through a special program at the university. We talk about music together, trading tunes on the piano once the house is clean. They live near the ocean in Brazil and have invited us to visit them when they return home. I'm planning on doing just that. I mean, *Por que não?*

9 Looking for Work

I've learned to survive and even thrive as a blind person, but, like other disabled people, I still face an uphill battle with potential employers. The experience I had when I lost my university job proved typical: as I mentioned, my boss had, in essence, fired me without having to tell me to my face. I had taken time off when I was first losing my sight. Later, when I met with her to discuss my return, she was evasive, never indicating that I couldn't return, but always suggesting that we wait a little longer. She put me off long enough to see that my contract lapsed and then simply didn't renew it. We never had an honest discussion about the situation. Because she never voiced her specific concerns, I had no chance to assuage them.

Until four years later, that is, when an opening in my old office was advertised in the local paper. It was for more or less my old position.

I had sought no legal remedy when my contract was terminated. With my confidence badly shaken (the newly disabled aren't exactly at the top of their self-esteem curves), I found myself wondering whether my old boss was right: perhaps I *couldn't* do the job, and I *would* embarrass myself and the office. Besides, I didn't care to work where I wasn't wanted.

Now things were different. Gus was in school and I was taking advantage of my newfound time, getting around town by foot, bus, or cab. I had my own talking computer. I had traveled independently—around the country and even overseas. My confidence was growing, as was my eagerness to get on with my life.

Resentment over my termination had grown, too, but by the time Mike and I visited an attorney, too much time had passed for us to take legal action. "But if a job ever comes open in that office," he counseled, "apply and see what happens." If I was offered employment, I could assume my boss had overcome her fear of disabilities. "If not, come and see me again."

In truth, I didn't want to sue. I just wanted my job back. And I wanted . . . "closure," maybe; or the simple pleasure of forcing my old boss to come clean. Since my résumé and cover letter outlined work experience that precisely matched the job description, the outside search committee took note. I was called for an interview.

Still using my white cane back then, I practiced walking the route. On the appointed day I arrived comfortably early and brimming with confidence. A former coworker greeted me and showed me to the conference room—but she wasn't on the search committee. In fact, I knew none of the people who faced me.

I met the committee members, shook hands with each, and slid gracefully into place. For fifteen minutes I fielded nuts-and-bolts questions about my qualifications and experience. Finally somebody broke the ice.

"Your résumé mentions that you've been trained to use a computer with speech synthesis. Can you tell us how that works?"

I explained about my IBM machine and the gates flew open; now they had permission to ask questions about blindness. How did I travel? Read books? Take notes? Everyone seemed very curious and sincerely interested; the interview was relaxed and friendly. I had thought a lot about how I would manage my duties without being able to see, and the committee seemed to appreciate my preparation. When the hour was up, everyone shook my hand again. One woman even patted me on the back and told me how impressed she was. It was no surprise when I received a letter inviting me to interview with the office staff.

——— ———

At the second interview, I knew every questioner. I had worked with all of them before. "Tell us a little about your relevant experience," one began.

So this is how it's going to be, I thought. They knew my work history as well as I did. But they asked, so I told them. In detail.

I heard pens on paper and pages shuffling as I talked, but no one interrupted with questions. When I finished, another voice piped up. "Now we're going to ask how you'd respond to certain situations. Let's say a parent calls from overseas, says her daughter has phoned her crying and wants to come home. . . ." One after another, such hypothetical situations were introduced. I responded sincerely, though it was hard to stop my jaw from dropping. These people had all witnessed how I'd responded to precisely these situations.

My ex-boss had been silent. She no doubt thought this session was as ludicrous as I did, but for different reasons. Although I couldn't see her, I knew she was crossing and uncrossing her legs, looking out the window, eager to conclude this charade. I was wasting her time—she'd decided that years ago.

"What about traveling?" she finally blurted out.

At last, I thought, knowing that the real question was "How can a blind person possibly travel overseas?" I turned toward her. (Even blind, I've always been good at facing people when they speak, and it can unnerve them.)

"I've been to Germany already since losing my sight," I answered confidently, "and I've traveled around the United States." I couldn't help thinking about that conference she'd denied me.

"Traveling is actually one of the easier things for me," I continued, knowing they might be as surprised to learn this as I had been. "Flight attendants are accommodating, and I always arrange to be met at the airport. I think this could be arranged on overseas visits as well. It's just a matter of preparation."

She was unmoved. "Well, maybe in the United States and in Germany, but what about other countries? We're hoping to start an exchange with Singapore. Do you know how people with handicaps are treated in Singapore?"

I had no idea.

"And how about those Australians?" she asked me. "They can be very brash."

I couldn't imagine how to answer that.

Then there was this: she was concerned that I wouldn't be able to walk fast enough. "You'd have to tour various foreign universities. I'm not sure you'd be able to keep up." I told her that I had been trained in "sighted guide," walking alongside a sighted companion, and that I could keep up very well this way.

"And how would you be able to tell whether or not people were lying to you in a meeting if you couldn't see their faces?"

"To be honest, I've never been good at that—sighted or blind."

My words faded into the ensuing silence, along with any lingering doubt about whether I actually wanted the job.

I didn't get the pleasure of turning it down. A few weeks later I received a rejection letter that cited, among other things, the fact that my experience wasn't sufficiently current. I decided against any legal follow-up. I was disgusted with those people by then; having dragged them as far as the interview process would have to suffice.

Unfortunately, in the dozen or so years since then, I've learned that this kind of experience is more rule than exception. On the face of it, things may appear (to the able-bodied world, at least) to have improved. Since passage of the Americans with Disabilities Act in 1990, the accessibility of public spaces has continued to improve. But of course bigotry is not abolished by curb cuts or audible "Walk" signals. As other minority groups have discovered, it's one thing to change laws; it's something else to change hearts and minds.

Some months ago I applied for a job with an emergency hotline that takes calls from people whose pets have eaten a toxic substance. I e-mailed for details, not mentioning my blindness. The e-mailed response enthusiastically suggested that I visit the office to apply.

The job required phone and computer work, according to the e-mail. Phones and computers are good tools for me: phones for obvious reasons, and computers because any common PC or Mac can be equipped with speech capabilities. *When I get to the interview,* I figured, *I'll even offer to pay for the adaptive software.*

A friend drove me to the office and helped me complete the printed application form. As we worked, I was aware of hushed, angst-ridden conversation in the background. The receptionist came and went; another woman emerged from the back room, disappeared again, then returned and, without so much as greeting me, launched into a shrill speech.

"Now, the problem is, when you take calls you have to fill out forms documenting everything."

I explained about talking computers. I could create digital versions of the forms, which I could complete and then print.

"No, they're legal forms that must be filled out by hand. We're in the process of computerizing and hope to be done in a few months, but right now it just won't work."

I tried to squeeze out more details to see if there were workarounds, and to address any other fears and concerns, but she wouldn't budge.

A few months later Mike spotted the very same ad in the paper again. I e-mailed the same contact; this time, no response. Weeks later a letter arrived—worded with extreme care, enumerating specific tasks described so as to leave no doubt that a blind person couldn't handle them. The product of a legal consultation, I was sure.

And all this for a part-time job. Eight dollars an hour.

It's hard to believe that legally acceptable accommodations couldn't have been made, allowing the completion of forms by computer. Especially in light of ADA. (Never mind that it would also have been more efficient.) But like my earlier boss, the woman at the poison center saw a blind person, a passel of problems, a situation she hoped would vanish quickly. I have experienced such treatment more times than I care to tell about. I don't take it as personally as I once did, but each time it's still painful and confounding.

Not that I can't understand how potential employers might be skeptical. It's easy for them to wonder what special arrangements would have to be made, and what it would cost. So every time I apply for a job, I struggle with whether to say, up front, that I'm blind. It's not something I can hide, or would care to—and I certainly don't want a potential employer to feel ambushed if the process leads to an interview. But when I *do* mention it at the outset, employers are free to imagine the worst, to build a case against me without ever sitting down with me.

All I want is a fair chance to learn about a job in detail and discuss how things might be worked out. In this regard, I sometimes wonder if the ADA hasn't further disadvantaged the disabled. It was intended to open doors; has it, instead, made prospective employers leery of litigation? Instead of hiring attorneys to craft job descriptions and bong letters, I'd much prefer employers to put all that energy into talking with me. Because I know, first hand, how things *can* work.

My first job as a blind person came as something of an accident. When Gus was an infant, my sister Cheryl introduced me to a friend whose eight-year-old daughter had multiple disabilities. One of the first questions Cheryl's friend asked was, "Do you go to church?"

Oh no, I thought. *She's going to tell me these children are God's angels or something.*

I'm sure that sounds harsh, but by then I'd heard an encyclopedia's worth of trite little statements from religious types:

"God never gives you something you can't handle."

"The Lord works in mysterious ways."

"Everything happens for a reason."

And my personal favorite: "God gives special children only to special parents."

Such folks often seemed to be trying to comfort themselves, not us. Rarely did I hear these platitudes from other blind people or from parents of handicapped kids.

But I needn't have worried about Cheryl's friend. Whatever her spiritual beliefs, she had a very practical motive for attending church: "Day to day, I can't always recognize the progress my daughter makes. But the people who see my daughter week to week at church have gotten to know her, to accept her. They see things I miss."

It made perfect secular sense to me, and so did introducing Gus to a community that was likely to accept him, no questions asked. I decided to give church a try.

I grew up a Lutheran but hadn't attended church regularly in years. So I thought I'd shop around. As it happened, the first church I visited was McKinley Presbyterian on the university campus. It had earned a reputation for putting its money and efforts where its religious mouth was; the sermon that Sunday confirmed this for me. A slide show depicted a recent construction project the church had helped sponsor, at a Down Syndrome institute in the Yucatan Peninsula. *Here's a church where Gus and I might fit in,* I realized immediately.

When it came time for the church's yearly fund raising phonathon, I signed up. Another volunteer read names and numbers onto a tape. We figured out other workarounds where necessary, and I raised money with the best of them. It wasn't work per se, but it was a confidence builder, a model of sorts.

My ears perked up one Sunday when someone announced that the church was looking for a part-time coordinator of volunteers. During the sermon I contemplated whether I could do the job. By the final "Amen," I'd decided to apply. But I didn't want my hiring to be a do-gooder thing. And I didn't want my bosses—the co-pastors of the church—to feel cornered. If they had gripes, if problems arose, I wanted them to tell me. So, during my interview, I suggested a sort of probation period: "If it isn't working for you after three months, I'll quit."

The job requirements were minimal. There were only two things I absolutely had to accomplish: get ushers for each service, and find someone to prepare the communion bread. How I filled the extra time was up to me, but I was to put in ten hours a week.

I started by having a volunteer read the church directory on tape. I entered the names and numbers into my computer so I could work at home. I had a desk and telephone at the church office, too; I'd bring the recorded directory and my cassette player when I wanted to call from there. I phoned everyone in the directory to introduce myself, using the opportunity to ask if there were volunteer jobs that especially interested them. With the large congregation, this project alone took many ten-hour weeks. Along the way I learned that the church had scads of committees. I began attending their monthly meetings and helped them find volunteers for their projects.

I was an ambitious, diligent, and productive worker. All parties were happy after three months, so I continued. Then an intern coordinator position came open at the foundation associated with the church. It involved working with college students, something I had enjoyed and was good at. And the fact that it was with the foundation, not the church, made me more comfortable—in truth, I've never been all that religious, at least in a conventional sense.

The job involved recruiting and supervising interns to work at the foundation's various endeavors, which included a seasonal shelter for the homeless, a second-hand clothing exchange, a food pantry for the poor, an art gallery, and a campus coffee shop. Most of the interns were sociology majors and future Peace Corps workers, but when we created a Saturday night music series in the coffee shop, advertising and commerce majors applied to gain hands-on experience in launching a new venture. Worlds collided as the socially conscious interns mixed with the commerce-minded résumé-builders. I enjoyed it all. I mediated their disputes and served as kind of an ad hoc counselor. It's cliché, but I've found that students mostly want someone to talk to without fear of ridicule. Only occasionally did they require pointed advice; mostly it was a matter of helping them herd their thoughts in one direction or another.

I had a very successful run in that position. It removed any remaining doubts I had about working, and it was terrific to be out there contributing to the well-being of others. But by the time Spyglass asked Mike to move up north to the new corporate office, I was ready for a change.

———

For several months settling into our new suburban digs took most of my time and energy. Once we'd established a routine, I found myself yearning to get out of the house while Gus was at school.

Since I needed to be home when Gus returned from school each day, I limited my job search to part-time work. As it happened, our town had a popular minor league baseball team, the Kane County Cougars. I learned that the team had an opening for someone to answer the phone, route calls, and take ticket orders.

The staff was young—for most it was their first job out of college. They were refreshingly unimpressed by my blindness, game to talk about the job and how I could manage it. We quickly discovered a problem: their phone system used lights to indicate which line was ringing. Unfazed, they agreed to let me have someone from the local Department of Rehabilitation Services office visit.

As helpful now as they had been years earlier (in my days at Braille Jail), DORS said the Cougars would have to install an entirely new phone system. The agency might be able to offer some financial assistance, but they could promise nothing until *after* I was hired. (Even today this policy continues, a Catch-22.)

While we were trying to sort this out, the staff had me come in a few times to make outgoing calls, the kind of calls they hated making—contacting groups who hadn't paid up, or soliciting schools to participate in special promotions. I didn't much like making these calls, either, but I figured it was a fair bargain.

We never did solve the original phone problem. Instead, the Cougars kept giving me more outgoing calls. I helped the group sales office to expand the school program. All in all, it was a terrific experience, another model for how, with a little patience and very little fanfare, these things can work. (Free game tickets were a fun perk.)

So, to that point, the scoreboard read 2-2: two good experiences (McKinley Presbyterian, Kane County Cougars), two bad (University of Illinois, poison hotline). There's one more, but it doesn't fit neatly in either category.

Much as I liked the Cougars job, I eventually got the itch for something different. I was reluctant to press for a full-time position because Mike and I weren't exactly committed to staying in the suburbs—from the start, we'd treated it as kind of a military posting.

I learned of a local hospice program that was seeking volunteers. I had some vaguely related experience, having been a crisis hotline volunteer back in Champaign. Since hospice would likewise involve counseling and matching resources to needs, I signed up for the training. It went splendidly. The agency seemed thrilled to have Dora and me at the weekly sessions; they proudly introduced us to visitors, practically making us the poster children for the volunteer program.

Only after I graduated did the trouble start. The training had been intense enough to create something of a bond among our volunteer group, so I'd kept in close touch with others. Soon every volunteer in our group had been assigned a patient—except me. When I called the agency to remind them that I was still available, they joked about the good news: there weren't enough people dying, so they couldn't assign me a case.

Months later, a friend from the class told me she was now seeing two patients. This time when I called, the agency admitted their reluctance. Dora's presence might bother a patient, they said, or I might inadvertently knock over bedside medications. "We have a patient now whom we considered assigning to you, Beth, but he sleeps on an air mattress. How would you be able to tell when the mattress needed more air?" I calmly reminded them that I still possessed my sense of touch.

Then came the classic, uncomfortably familiar line: "Really, it's not us. We're just afraid the families will have a problem with you."

Yeah, and Americans might be all right with disabled people, but those Australians, whew, they can really be brash.

I asked if they'd be more comfortable if I didn't work directly with the hospice patient. "How about if I limit myself to counseling the patients' family and friends?"

"I don't know, Beth," the hospice woman said. "We're just afraid the families might see you as needier than they are."

A decade earlier I'd have cradled my head in my hands and cried, looked for comfort from Mike. But ten years of blindness had taught me how to stand up to ignorance and small-mindedness. I stayed on this agency's case, phoning weekly to remind them that I remained available. I regularly attended educational meetings and even had a reunion party at our house for everyone who had graduated from our training course.

The agency eventually gave in.

Ernie, my first hospice patient, was an uncommunicative and eccentric old coot. None of his friends or family was willing to take care of him at home, so when his cancer got bad enough, he was forced to check into a local nursing home. "We usually don't send volunteers to nursing homes," the volunteer coordinator told me. "But the home called asking for someone. Apparently Ernie won't talk to them about dying. Actually, he won't talk to them about *anything.*" Other volunteers had turned down this assignment.

I visited Ernie three times a week. At first I did all the talking, but after a few weeks he finally tired of listening and began to speak up. By the end of two months together, Ernie and I had hatched a plan to rent a wheelchair so that I could push him onto one of the local riverboat casinos. I'd never been gambling, and he wanted to show me how. Sadly, we never got our chance, but before he was transferred to intensive care at the hospital, he let me hold his hand. Dora and I were given family status at the ICU and allowed to see Ernie as often as we wanted. Mike came with me and Dora to Ernie's wake.

I was assigned other cases after that, often "problem cases" that other volunteers didn't want. For instance, the African-American woman who was caring for her dying father on the tough side of neighboring Aurora. I didn't mind. I got to know a wonderful woman whose path I would never have crossed otherwise. She invited Dora and me to attend her church with her; when we did, we were treated like royalty.

On balance, I have to put my hospice experience in the plus column. I played by the rules, encountered resistance, and overcame it with persistence. Ultimately I demonstrated I could do the work. In addition, hospice helped me understand my own life. I realized that losing my sight bore a certain similarity to losing a loved one. When someone dear to you dies, you're badly shaken and you miss them. Over time you grow used to their absence, but the background ache never vanishes completely. And you can be cruising along just fine when, out of the blue, something reminds you of your loss and you grieve all over again.

That's how it's been with my eyesight. I'm accustomed to being blind now, and I can go for weeks without thinking much about it. But then old footage of the Beatles will appear on TV, or I'll put one of my shirts through the whole laundry cycle with an untreated stain on it. The floodgates open. To this day I'm astounded by how the smallest things generate the greatest sadness. In the past, applying for work could be such a trigger. I'd be reminded of losing my old job, and soon I'd find myself wondering what I might be doing if I could still see. I'd get angry. I'd resent having to talk my way into positions for which I was overqualified. I'd find myself wonder why things have to be so damn hard.

It's not as bad now—these feelings seem to recede as fast as they wash over me. But it's still tough. Each time I consider applying for a job, I weigh whether it's worth the trouble, and not just because I might encounter resistance—also because I might lose my disability benefits. If I earn too much, I become ineligible. It's not that I worry about losing the stipend, but I cannot afford to endanger the health insurance. Between Gus and me, our little family isn't the kind of risk insurers willingly assume. That makes this a high-stakes game: if I take a shot at a job that ultimately fizzles, we could find ourselves in a world of trouble.

Yet, if the right chance comes along, I'll gladly take that risk. Meanwhile, I piece together interesting bits of work. After my disappointment with the poison hotline, for example, I was feeling a little down until I heard that the art department on campus needed nude models.

Back when I was a sighted undergraduate, I wouldn't have

dreamed of trekking across campus to disrobe in front of a roomful of other students. To this day I still undress behind a closed door. But now, when I walk with Dora, I'm sure that every eye is on us. Could it be OK for people to watch me, as long as that's what they're *assigned* to do? I had to find out.

At the informational meeting I felt as though I had died and gone to blind job-seeking heaven—they badly needed models, and my eyesight was a complete non-factor. The only bothersome comment came when I had to admit that I'd just turned forty. The interviewer mentioned that it would be nice to have a middle-aged model.

I let the comment slide. If they wanted a middle-aged model, I'd be a middle-aged model.

On the first day the instructor was particularly pleased that I brought Dora along. "The students can draw both of you. And since you'll be there with the dog," she reasoned, "we'll have you keep your dress on."

Modeling was an interesting enough experience that I kept a journal about it. Eventually I turned my entries into an essay that was published in the local weekly alternative newspaper and later picked up by a national wire service. I've written regularly for the weekly ever since, and have even published a story or two in national magazines. I enjoy the writing itself, but the research and reporting aspects are even better. That's what gets me out into the community, doing what I like best: meeting new people and talking with them about their lives.

I've gradually become a public speaker. Dora and I make the rounds, from elementary schools to nursing homes. As you might guess, Dora is a big hit—sometimes I think they'd be just as happy to have her back without me. I don't mind; I've become something of an unofficial ambassador for The Seeing Eye.

Lately I've made it a personal priority to talk about employment issues. One of my newspaper stories covered the working blind in our local communities; after that, I was invited onto a radio talk show. I'm working this into the talks I give at service clubs—the Rotary, Lions, and so on. I've spoken to these groups for years; they're always gracious and glowingly appreciative, but I wonder how they'd respond if I walked into their businesses and applied for a job. And that's my message these days: "If you're impressed with my courage and my resourcefulness, just imagine what kind of employee I'd be."

I like my work life as it is right now, the writing and speaking. But I'd drop it in a New York minute if one of the folks I spoke to offered me a full time position; one like the job I had back when I could see. All I need is for someone to meet me halfway. It hasn't happened yet, but I'm still looking.

Epilogue

After I'd first returned home with Pandora, I twice phoned The Seeing Eye to send someone out to help us. The first time was after Pandora (nicknamed Dora by then) decided she didn't want to work. On a sultry summer morning we had taken only one step out onto the porch when she crouched down, refusing to move. "You know, you're right!" I told her. "It's too hot for a walk." We turned around and went back inside.

From that day forward, whatever the weather, Dora tested me. I'd pick up her harness and command, "Forward!" She wouldn't budge, crouching on the sidewalk instead. I'd go into my regular routine, using all the leash corrections I'd been taught. We'd eventually get going, only to repeat the same scene a few blocks farther along, then again.

The visiting field representative from The Seeing Eye first tightened Dora's collar. "Maybe now she'll actually feel your leash corrections!" he laughed. I was shown how to tighten the collar around her ears right from the start of our walks, told not to loosen it until she was trotting at a good pace. He also showed me a different way to hold the harness and leash, a style that would constantly remind Dora that I was back there, wanting to move along.

The second visit came years later, when Dora began slowing down in the middle of intersections. It made me nervous when we were on busy streets; I was afraid that the light would change and we'd get hit.

"She's anticipating the stop she has to make at the up curb," the visiting field rep explained. "So she starts slowing down in the middle of the street to get ready to stop."

The Seeing Eye taught dogs to stop at every curb, whether down or up. The field rep suggested I quit requiring Dora to stop at the up curbs, and to praise her lavishly once she made the step up. It worked. Dora started hurrying across the streets just to earn my praise for crossing successfully.

Dora never did become a speedy dog. Given her druthers, she would always choose hanging out at home instead of working. That said, for eleven years she kept me safe on the streets, guided me through office buildings and shopping malls, traveled with me on buses, trains, and airplanes. At eight years old, she developed arthritis in her shoulder. Daily aspirin helped, and she continued working. After her twelfth birthday her pace slowed enough to convince me to retire her. I could have decided to keep her. But when a nearby friend agreed to adopt her, I made arrangements to return to The Seeing Eye for a new dog in November, 2001.

Dora rode with us the morning Mike drove me to the airport. "You'll have fun living with Randy," I assured her, giving her a final hug. I managed not to cry.

The commuter flight was late into O'Hare; I'd missed my connection. The redcap left me at a phone—I needed to call The Seeing Eye to say I'd be late. Phone call completed, I absentmindedly leaned down to pick up Dora's harness. The tears finally came.

A lot had changed at The Seeing Eye. We were no longer formally addressed by our last names, and the dress code was much more liberal: instead of requiring dresses and suit jackets at lunchtime, they simply "requested" no jeans or sweatpants. A new dormitory wing had been added, which meant students had private rooms, rather than roommates.

Another significant change: we had to wait two days before meeting our new dogs. "We want to get to know you as best we can before matching you with a dog," my trainer explained.

I spent those first two days either stumbling around with my cane or walking with Robert, my assigned trainer. He even drove me to downtown Morristown for a "Juno Walk": he held the front of the harness, I held the back, and he led me around town. "Tell me if I'm walking too fast or too slow," he instructed. "I want to get a feel for your pace."

My class had twenty students. Each of us, it turned out, had worked with a Seeing Eye dog before. Dinner conversation centered on dogs, and as in any group, individuals quickly assumed their roles: the Expert, the Victim, the Whiner, the Jokester.

I remained uncharacteristically quiet. I loved Dora, but I was still no dog lover. Glimmers of my former Seeing Eye experience returned. *If I speak, I might be busted, exposed as the non–dog lover of this group.*

Each of the four trainers had five students. For the first week we five sat together with him at meals. The Expert was assigned to Robert's group with me, as well as Me Too Woman, who needed to have done anything anyone else in the group had done. (I'd had some articles published; she was a writer, too. I modeled nude for art students; so did she.) With Me Too Woman seated on one side and the Expert on the other, there was no reason for me to say a word.

At a private interview on my first night, Robert asked, "Is there a certain breed, a certain gender you need?" I didn't know what to say. My real concern was getting a dog with a good name. The puppies in each litter born at The Seeing Eye are given names that start with the same letter. Pandora was from the "P" litter, for example. To avoid repeating names too often, The Seeing Eye sometimes gets overly creative (rather like the folks who name hurricanes). I didn't know what might happen to my self-respect if my dog bore the name Bouquet, or Gremlin, or Yorba.

My need for a well-named dog seemed too juvenile to admit. "No," I finally answered. "I'll take whatever you think is best." As Robert stood up to leave, I added, "I really would like a faster dog this time, though."

Be careful what you wish for. My new dog is a one-year-old yellow ball of energy, a cross between a golden retriever and Labrador retriever. As I write this, it's amazing to think we've only been home together for a month; she is extremely attached to me, and I already feel tremendously confident with her. She loves to work, often nudging my wrist as I sit at the computer. *Can't we go outside yet?*

———   ——

Our walks must look comical—she pulls with such enthusiasm that curbs seem to surprise her. She stops, but often not until the last millisecond. I imagine us in a Hanna-Barbera cartoon, the sound of my rubber soles squealing on the pavement, sparks shooting out behind my heels at every stop. Her tail stands straight up as she works, and I often find myself laughing with joy at her exuberance.

The only thing I struggle with is—surprise—her name. Three dogs assigned to our class were born in the "H" litter. Her brothers had great names: Homer, Herbie. Their sister was less fortunate.

"Honey. That's nice," I said to Robert when he introduced us. I was already on the floor with my new dog, rubbing her belly.

"Not Honey," he said. "*Hah*nee."

"Huh? I furrowed my eyebrows. "How do you spell it?"

"H-a-n-n-i. Pretend you're from Alabama and you're saying 'Honey.'"

I scratched Hanni's ears, and she sprung up to kiss me. OK, I smiled. I can live with the name.

At dinner, Me Too Woman reported that her dog, too, had kissed her when they met. "Mine has an odd name, too," she added. The expert cut in, warning us of the dangers in changing a Seeing Eye dog's name.

Thank goodness we each had our own dorm room. Mine provided a refuge, and it allowed one-on-one time with Hanni. I regretted not having spent enough time early on bonding with Dora. I was determined things would go differently now, and they did.

The decision to learn with a new Seeing Eye dog is rather like the decision to update a computer and its software. Often the old computer still works fine; it's just too slow, or isn't capable of a few functions you think would be handy. You know that learning a new computer and new programs is going to be a pain. You'll be clumsy at first. It's frustrating, but you know that if all goes well, you'll end up with a faster machine, one more reliable and with more capabilities.

And so it was with Hanni.

Over the years, Dora had become so slow that I was unconsciously pushing her along, rather than letting her pull me. Hanni didn't like this behavior on my part. It confused her—she was supposed to pull me, and I wasn't letting her. Robert tightened Hanni's harness in a way that made it difficult for me to lift it and push, and on our routes through Morristown he kept a close eye on me, scolding and coaching me to keep the harness where it belonged. It reminded me of piano lessons, with teachers struggling to rid me of the bad techniques I'd developed after years of playing on my own.

I didn't battle Robert, and I wasn't defensive. This time I just wanted to hone my technique. Getting proper harness placement was key to my success with Hanni, and after a few days it was easy. Whenever I held the harness correctly, she flew. We skated down the sidewalks of Morristown, narrowly avoiding parking meters, garbage cans, telephone poles. "I don't have any fingernails left!" Robert laughed after following us on one trip.

Hanni and I were often paired up with John, a computer programmer, and Rudy, his German shepherd. Me Too Woman sometimes came along. In addition to the Me-Too thing, she was chronically late. John and I would often sit belted in the van while Robert ran back to the dorm to fetch her.

So it was on the day of my epiphany. John and I were laughing in the back of the van when Me Too Woman (Sarah was her name) arrived. We heard her command "Forward!"; we heard her dog jump in; then we heard her slide off the step and fall onto the pavement.

John and I went immediately silent. She was sobbing. I felt helpless, as if the seatbelt couldn't be unbuckled for me to get out to help her. But really, it was the blindness, and the dogs at our feet, that kept us from jumping up. Robert was there in an instant. Sarah got up, assured her dog that she was all right, and somehow managed to get herself into the van. I heard her pull out a tissue to dry her eyes.

Every blind person has been in that situation: falling, running into a wall, making a mistake in public. Most of us hate being pitied by those who witness our mishaps. John and I continued to remain silent. Once she had fastened her seatbelt, Robert explained our route for the day. John and I asked questions; she drove with us to town and worked with her dog like everyone else.

I was ashamed of myself for how I'd been responding to my fellow students, especially to Sarah and the Expert. (She had a name, too: Ruth.) It took Sarah's fall for me to realize that these women didn't need an attitude adjustment—*I* did. It's not easy being blind. We'd all been through hell in one way or another.

At dinner that night I asked Sarah what she liked to write about. "Science fiction," she said. She'd written a couple of screenplays for TV but had never submitted them. We talked about whom she might contact, where she could get help.

The next morning Ruth was in the van with us. John had gone on a solo trip, leaving Ruth and me alone to talk. When I asked about her childhood, I found out she had been born blind and had attended special schools. "The kids in my neighborhood all called me 'Dummy,'" she said matter-of-factly. "They thought just because I was blind, I was stupid." Ruth was about my age, had a government job, lived in her own apartment, and was very involved with her church.

Many other people in our class were also churchgoers. One arranged to have the Christian band she played in perform for us the next Saturday. Earlier I had decided not to go—I didn't want anyone getting the idea I was interested in evangelism. But after Sarah's fall, I was feeling more generous. I attended the concert, and although I didn't agree with the message, the music was top-notch. By chance, I sat next to a lawyer from Toronto, the only student in our class whose dog had a name stranger than Hanni's. I'd already met Vogler but hadn't yet had a chance to speak with his human, Richard. We hit it off right away, and I still correspond with him via e-mail.

After the concert we all took our dogs to the park, and then I joined in on something else I'd heretofore shunned: karaoke. For this, I needed a beer. Jerry, a retired cafeteria manager and vending machine operator, had a supply and was happy to oblige. The music started; the microphone traveled between evangelists and beer drinkers. Aside from the couple of dogs who groaned in protest at sour notes, we all had a great time.

At Braille Jail I'd done everything I could to avoid being grouped with "those blind people." Without realizing it, I had still been resisting when I arrived at The Seeing Eye, even the second time around. How foolish. I thrive on meeting and talking to people—I'll listen to anyone who's willing to talk about their struggles, their worries, their hopes. Had I stayed aloof, what an opportunity I might have missed.

Still, the final few days away from home seemed to drag on. I was elated on the December afternoon when Hanni and I finally set foot into Champaign's small terminal.

Mike watched us from the other side of the security checkpoint. "She's *fast!*" he exclaimed. "You guys were a blur!" He welcomed me with a long embrace, a kiss, and an expression of relief that I was back. He'd missed me, and he was worn out from being a single parent for three weeks. He'd done it before, of course, when I got Pandora. But, as he likes to say, he's getting older, and Gus is getting bigger.

The first time I went to The Seeing Eye, Mike had started a new job shortly before I left. Likewise the second time. After years of technical writing and marketing communications jobs, he decided to try out newspaper writing. Last year he received his master's degree in journalism at the University of Illinois; already he's senior editor of the local weekly.

I had arranged for special education students from the university to take Gus off the bus every day while I was away, but it was just Mike and Gus the rest of the time. Dad was ready for a break.

Now that I'm back, I do my part with Gus again, juggling care for him with daily walks and continued training with Hanni. After the Christmas and New Year's holidays, we all seem to have settled into our routines. Gus attends school. I write every morning. With book revisions finished now, I'll start on a story assignment from a national magazine.

I enjoy freelance writing. I'm gradually picking up more work, and my disability simply isn't an issue; my work is appreciated for its own sake. And I get to set my own schedule. My volunteer work for hospice continues, and I've developed a specialization in grief and bereavement. I regularly visit a woman with multiple sclerosis whose husband/caretaker died last year, and I help facilitate a support group for those who have recently lost loved ones.

My work as a nude model is increasing, too. I have modeled for the university and for private studios, and I'm about to debut at the local community college. Dora was good at modeling: dignified, poised, and largely immobile. I miss her, but I haven't yet gone to visit at her new home. I want to give her time to bond with Randy, her new owner.

"Ah, she's doing great!" Randy exclaimed. The first day he went to work after her arrival, he put some stuff on the couch. "You know, so Dora wouldn't get up there while I was away."

He needn't have done that, I thought. *Dora never climbs onto furniture.*

When he came home for lunch that day, Dora had dragged everything off the couch. "There she was, nestled in the pillows," Randy laughed. "All she had up there with her was the TV remote control."

Sounds as though Dora is enjoying her retirement. She's probably happy to be have concluded her modeling career, too. No doubt Hanni will enjoy zipping me to my new gig—I'm curious to find out how long she can sit still.

Acknowledgments

First, I thank my handsome husband. Mike Knezovich helped write, edit, proofread, and revise each chapter of this book; only his generosity of spirit has kept his name from appearing on the title page along with mine. Mike says some day he might like to write a book of his own. I hope he will. He's a great writer.

If my family and friends weren't so much fun, it might have been difficult for me to ask them for all the assistance I needed with this project. My sister Cheryl photocopied, bound, and shipped each and every version. Ed Finke, Rick Amodt, and my sisters took photos and donated them to the cause, as did Jim Neill, Lois Haubold, and Gia Ciambotti. Steve Otto assembled the very first draft. Milton Otto and Carl Reisman provided valuable legal advice. Dr. Terry Ernest read over the medical bits to make sure I had them right. Jean Thompson, Theresa Miller, and Jane Lawrence edited some of the early drafts. Mary McHugh cheered me on at the end.

Special thanks go to those who voluntarily read the manuscript aloud so I could listen for errors: The Dare County Writers' Group, Brad Hudson, the Senese family, Keith Pickerel, Kevin Goldstein, Bonita Mall, and Audio Studio for the Reading Impaired, Inc.

The number of friends who agreed to read my manuscript (and suggest valuable changes) is so large that I cannot list all their names.

David Long and Rick Canning deserve special mention, however; this book absolutely would not have been the same without their help.

One of the luckiest days of my life was the day that Rick wrote Ann Lowry's name on a piece of paper and shoved it into my hand. Ann's encouragement was honest and unwavering; she's made *Long Time, No See* a much better book than the 700-page saga I dropped on her desk years ago. My thanks go to her and her colleagues at the University of Illinois Press.

Thanks, finally, to Gus. He sat on my lap and laughed as I typed the first draft on my talking computer. He and the manuscript shared my attention during years of revision. And right now, though he wants me to turn over the cassette in his tape player, he waits patiently for me to finish this page. He's a good guy.

Beth Finke is a freelance writer and part-time nude model for art classes in Urbana, Illinois. Her articles have been published in *Writer Magazine,* the *Anchorage Press, The Bark,* and *Dog Fancy,* and she appears as a commentator on National Public Radio's "Morning Edition."

The University of Illinois Press
is a founding member of the
Association of American University Presses.

Composed in 10.5/14 Minion
with Triplex display
by Barbara Evans
at the University of Illinois Press
Designed by Paula Newcomb
Manufactured by Thomson-Shore, Inc.

University of Illinois Press
1325 South Oak Street
Champaign, IL 61820-6903
www.press.uillinois.edu